THE POWER OF
INTERACTIVE CARE
THERE IS A BETTER WAY

Breaking the Mould of Traditional Disability Support

By Julienne Verhagen

First published by Busybird Publishing 2018

Copyright © 2018 Julienne Verhagen

ISBN 978 19 258 3018 7

Julienne Verhagen has asserted her right under the Copyright, Designs and Patents Act 1988 to be identified as the author of this work. The information in this book is based on the author's experiences and opinions. The publisher specifically disclaims responsibility for any adverse consequences, which may result from use of the information contained herein. Permission to use information has been sought by the author. Any breaches will be rectified in further editions of the book.

All rights reserved. No part of this publication may be reproduced, stored in or introduced into a retrieval system, or transmitted in any form, or by any means (electronic, mechanical, photocopying, recording or otherwise) without the prior written permission of the author. Any person who does any unauthorised act in relation to this publication may be liable to criminal prosecution and civil claims for damages. Enquiries should be made through the publisher.

Cover image: Julienne Verhagen

Cover design: Busybird Publishing

Layout and typesetting: Busybird Publishing

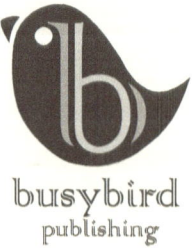

Busybird Publishing
2/118 Para Road
Montmorency, Victoria
Australia 3094
www.busybird.com.au

Dedication

To the amazing, high-quality carers we've had the privilege to work with, watching them take the greatest of care with my brother Scott. We are so, so grateful for your ingenuity, attention to detail, friendship, sense of fun, extraordinary positivity, intuitiveness and action. To so many of you, thank you for your authentic relationships with our Scotty, for your style and fun and for striving to make his family members welcome anytime. To the Damiens, the Robs and the Olivias of this world: we are so blessed to have had your expertise, service and friendship. You are the shining light in the lives of all the people you support.

To my mum, Sandra, for the courageous, compassionate act of taking on three children who weren't your own, with special needs, by choice. And for raising six kids, often on your own, while seeking new ways of thinking and trailblazing the way forward. Thank you for fighting the good fight to this day. For protecting, nurturing and adding value to all our lives.

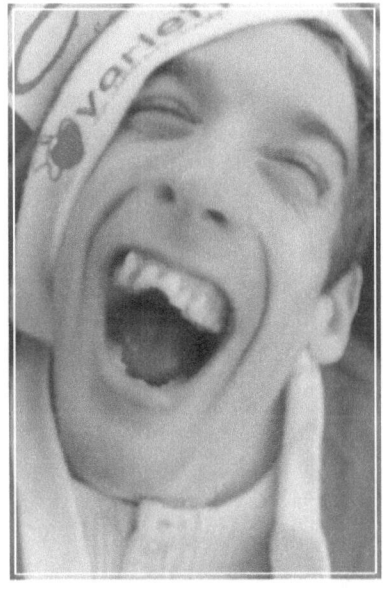

To my amazingly inspirational brother, Scott Clough: thank you for teaching everyone you meet about the essence of *you*. Your courage, your patience, your determination and your capacity to love and be joyous is not only infectious, it's instructional. Everyone around you feels your beautiful spirit, as you add humanity and humility to our fast-paced, self-indulgent world. Thank you for contributing to this book. Not only the text that you painstakingly wrote with your wonderful support workers to add your important voice to each chapter, but in no small way for your courage, your determination, your smiles and your indomitable spirit.

Thank you for giving all of us in our family a direction and an outlet to serve. Love ya buddy.

Contents

Introduction	1
Chapter 1 - Scotty and Me	5
Chapter 2 - Revolution? It's Time!	17
Chapter 3 - Choices, Choices, Choices	23
Chapter 4 - Horrors and Heroes	31
Chapter 5 - Embody Leadership Everyday	43
Chapter 6 - Boredom Kills – Everything	51
Chapter 7 - Safety! – With Life	61
Chapter 8 - No Institutionalised Insanity	73
Chapter 9 - Touchpoints of Care	85
Chapter 10 - Crucial, Meaningful Relationships	93
Chapter 11 - Support the Supporters!	105
Chapter 12 - Interactive Care Action	117
Afterword	121
Next Steps	123
About The Author	125
Work With Julienne	126
Workshops	127
Interactive Care Certification	129
Packages	131
Endnotes	133

Disclaimer

Purpose: The purpose of this book is to raise awareness about disability care. The statistics, examples and stories detailed are meant to highlight the relevant issues and come from my experience and perspective. I have tried to recreate events, locales and conversations from my own memories. Everything is how I remember it, and people might disagree, but these are my own memories, opinions and conclusions.

Names: In order to protect their privacy, I have changed the names of some individuals and places in my stories. I may have changed some identifying details such as physical characteristics, relationships, occupations and places of residence.

Variety: The stories in this book come from varied sources, organisations, places and times from my life and career, and are not necessarily focused on recent or current situations with myself or family members.

Julienne Verhagen

Introduction

Why write a book about changing the way people care for those with disabilities? Because, while most would agree we've come a long way, there is still much work to be done.

At academic, medical and advocacy conferences around the world, able-bodied people speak of funding models, treatments, United Nation conventions, anti-discriminatory laws and broad-based inclusion. And while all of these things are important, it doesn't seem to change the day-to-day experience of your child's life, if they rely on service providers and paid workers to help care for them.

Your wonderfully unique, precious person who is so important to you is actually quite vulnerable – to being undereducated, undernourished, bored, and damaged in their spirit. If they have limited mobility and limited or no speech, then to have any hope of an innovative, interesting, safe and meaningful life, they need you, their family and friends, to advocate for them.

You also need some awesome disability support workers – those who support their clients to live their lives with joy. Many of them do amazing work, reserving diligent, positive, intuitive attention for their clients, but many are simply not up to that standard.

How do you do this? How do you find the best support? What is reasonable to ask for and expect of activity centres, schools, respite care and group homes? Family members find themselves tirelessly advocating for their person with disability, not knowing which battles to fight and how to fight them – what's reasonable and what's totally impractical.

This book will be a guide for you.

I've written this with disability support workers and their managers in mind. My intention is to give simple, quick and affordable ways for support workers to improve job satisfaction in their roles, to hire (and fire) the right people so that you have support workers who have the right mindset – to be proactive, creative, empathetic – and find natural, fun and stimulating ways to be more interactive with our wonderful family members.

If you are a professional worker in this field, thank you for reading this book. Please note that while I do express my frustration at times, I have done your job and I've felt your frustrations. Chapter 11 is where I try to give balance to the picture. If you want to know how much I want to support you guys and change the culture of service providers from the inside out, you are welcome to jump ahead and read chapter 11 first!

If you are a support worker, primary carer or practitioner who feels critiqued by some of my ideas: just consider them food for thought. Every person with disability is different, every home situation is different and every support worker is different. I'm just trying to highlight areas that could easily be so much better for so many people. Please consider my points.

I want to acknowledge and praise the incredibly awesome disability support workers and family members out there who are fighting the good fight, creating change and doing their best with their wonderful clients and family members, day-in and day-out. I've taken the very best that I've seen, heard and experienced from you all and given it a descriptive name to encapsulate what great support really is. You see, I know there is a better way. I call it Interactive Care.

The self-advocacy movement, where people with disability who can speak up for themselves are being encouraged to do so, is making a real difference. Now we need the right people to listen!

Just a word about the language used in this book. Language shapes the way we view the world. The words we use can influence community perspectives and attitudes – and therefore can impact the lives of others. When we change how we write and speak about people with disability, we can profoundly change the way they are viewed by the community and even themselves.

There has been a strong movement in the field to stop labelling the disease or disability before the person, and person-first referencing has become the norm. This is not about political correctness but about being respectful to the person. Do we talk about Glasses-face Grace, Fat Freddy or Diabetes Diana? Of course not. So why do we still say Autistic Adam or Wheelchair-bound Wendy? We use person-first language now.

Most people with any sort of impairment have multiple 'disabilities', so it's no longer preferred to say, 'people with a disability', or 'people with disabilities', but to use the generalised 'people with disability'.

So, in a nutshell, I no longer say:

> 'My spastic and blind brother Scott, who is wheelchair-bound, and my step-brother Robby, who is mildly retarded, each suffer from being handicapped.'

Instead I now say:

> 'Scott is my brother, who has cerebral palsy, is visually impaired and uses a wheelchair, and Robby is my step-brother, who has a learning difficulty. They are both people with disability.'

To add to the confusion, it's not always the same in other countries. In the UK, for example, they still prefer the phrase 'disabled people', and in other countries there is a big push to use 'ability' language, rather than focusing on the limitations a person might face.

Got all that? No? I'm not surprised! I slip up from time to time too – but, most people with disability say that as long as you're putting the person first, and it's said with good intent, then you can't go too far wrong.

Some terms used in this book, for clarification and ease of writing:

NDIS:	National Disability Insurance Scheme.
Carer:	This term is being phased out in Australia, as historically it denotes a parent figure who makes decisions for and about the person. When I use it in this book, it's as a general term for someone who supports their person, whether it be a paid, unpaid, family or volunteer position.
Primary Carer:	A person (usually a family member) who is the person with disability's main person of support.
Practitioner:	Any medical, treatment or specialist professional who works with people with disability.
Self-advocate:	A person with disability who can and does make their wishes known.

Chapter 1

Scotty and Me

> *Hi, I'm Scott, and I have a lot to say! I'm very, very excited to contribute to this book and I'm proud of my big sis for putting her heart and soul into Interactive Care. I'm blind and I don't speak, but I can hear and understand you and I'd like to be friends.*
>
> *Who am I really? I'm smart – I remember everything! I'm the smiley guy. I love to laugh, and sing along to music, and clap my hands for 'yes'! I like to use my voice even though my body betrays my desire to speak words. I live in my head. I think all the time. I have feelings and dreams. I love my family and miss seeing them, but overall I'm a happy guy, a source being. I am me.*
>
> Scott Clough

Hello, and welcome to *The Power of Interactive Care*. It's my manifesto – and I can be pretty blunt about the way things are, good and bad and in between. It's time to 'get real' about the total joy that people with disability can experience, the terrible pain that they often go through, the achievements that are possible for them to accomplish, and the way to make that sort of magic happen.

This book is written for parents, family members and primary carers of a person with disability. Whether you have newly diagnosed child, a sibling who's school aged, a parent with a brain injury that you are learning to adjust to, or your adult son is now in care and you're dealing with a foreign world of frustration – this book is for you. It will highlight and forewarn about areas of frustration, pain and preventable distress.

I hope that self-advocates, people with disability, and their advocates will also gain from reading about common issues that are faced, and overcome, by others when the right mindset is applied to everyday situations.

For most of us, the journey into the world of disability was an unexpected one accompanied by fear, shock and overwhelm. What does this all mean? How did this happen? What am I in for? How will I cope? Will my loved one ever live a full and happy life?

I can't answer all of your questions, and I cannot give definite assurances – as

every person, every condition, every situation is different. Finding a helpful perspective though on what it can be like raising a child with disability can really change how we look at our situation.

There's a poem written by American author and social activist Emily Perl Kingsley, who has also been a writer for Sesame Street since 1970, that I find useful. She describes her experience having a child with autism (autism spectrum disorder) by using the metaphor of planning for a trip to France. You're all prepared and excited for your trip, but when the plane lands, the flight attendant says: 'Welcome to Holland!' You're shocked and dismayed, as you wanted to go to France – but in Holland you must now stay. The thing is you haven't been sent to somewhere horrible, dirty and disease-ridden; Holland is actually a beautiful place - with windmills, tulips and Rembrants' – it's just very different to France.

Not only can this metaphor for having a child with disability be apt, but, because my father was Dutch, Holland feels very much like home to me – it feels gezellig. And so does being around people with disability. I feel very comfortable in 'Holland'!

Many people find great comfort from this concept. Others find that having a child with disability is nothing like the serenity of Holland, but rather like being on a never-ending rollercoaster ride, or trekking through the jungle with no map. Whatever is it for you, I want to help you have the best quality support for your person with disability as possible; and give you some guide as to what it will take to make that happen.

The power of Interactive Care is that, using the eight themes of Interactive Care, most solutions to complex problems can be simple, easy, cheap and manageable.

They can create incredible changes in the quality of life for everyone – client, worker and family alike. If you're a family member of a person with disability, my great hope is that you'll pass this book on to their support workers (and their managers) to take that next step into improving their effectiveness, increasing job satisfaction and providing exceptional quality of support for the people they work for: the clients.

If you are a disability support worker: I know how terrific, and how tough, your job can be. There is much in here for you – not only insights from the family and client perspective, but ideas, resources, and a new perspective on many everyday occurrences, and how we can make small but significant differences immediately to improve our client's lives.

This is not meant to condemn anyone for what I see as wrong-doings of the past. It's not a blame game towards governments, parents who have put their children into institutions, misinformed doctors, or educators who judged intelligence and learning capability without a clue what they were really doing. This is not a finger-pointing exercise towards for those support workers I have experienced who are not up to standard, or integration-aids, nurses, or aged-care workers. All 'carers' rely on training, modelling, leadership, budgets and workplace culture to do a job well, and they have no real influence in a vacuum.

This book is a wake-up call, parallel to and in alignment with the NDIS, fee-for-service, the #Metoo campaign, the Royal Commission into Institutional Responses to Child Sexual Abuse, and contemporary 21st century community values. This is our opportunity to make things better. It's time. As Maya Angelou said:

> *Do the best you can until you know better. Then when you know better, do better.*

Whether you feel that all institutions, group homes, banal sheltered workshops and boring activity centres need to be completely re-thought and closed forever (which will take time to achieve), or you believe these places can be effective and inclusive if just managed from a different perspective, I'm here to say that we can make lives better now. We can improve many living situations for people with disability – immediately.

And the solutions are not usually difficult or expensive to begin; they come from a perspective of common sense aligned with the best intent for the client. I'm not asking for huge, unrealistic, ground-breaking change here. I want to show that with a little thoughtfulness and a positive mindset, great things can happen. Add good immersive training and excellent leadership, and just about anything is possible!

For those changes that are more difficult and might require political discussion, changes in legislation or re-working of company policies – let's start that conversation. (Laws and policies change all the time – when the community demand action.)

As family members, navigating either a new or a well worn path to daily life for our person with disability can seem overwhelming like a minefield. Paths we've done one hundred times before now have landmines! Sometimes we see a tiny little track detour, and by following it we discover a whole new vista that can open up our world. It's rare that we get a view to see where we're going, or even where we've been – but one thing is sure – you just have to keep walking. If you're in the same situation, keep asking questions, keep up with current resources, and keep loving your child/nephew/sister/grandparent/family friend all you can.

Sometimes it's about working smarter rather than harder. Taking hold of the reins in some areas, and loosening them off in other areas.

With the NDIS coming in to Australia, there is more opportunity to have choice of support. If you're hiring your own carers, choosing wisely (knowing what to look for, ask them and expect from them) will make all the difference in your stress levels and their lives. Knowing your rights within a service provider will help to know what's reasonable to ask for; accessing the amazing array of support groups, websites and resources in the community can help give your person with disability so many more activities, options and opportunities than you might otherwise have realised.

That then means you can loosen the reins on always being the primary carer, housecleaner, taxi driver, finance manager and spokesperson for your person with disability. You can start having a life too!

And I don't mean this comment flippantly. You having a life – both with your person with disability and as your own person – is the joy that we do all of this for. Getting the right standard of care in place, whenever and wherever you can, not only give them a better life, but you and your family as well.

Parents are always thinking, 'Have we done enough?' Yes, things can get tiring and the fight for better equipment, rights, education, access and inclusion can really wear you down. Many of us get caught up in the cycle of one situation requiring advocacy, after the next after the next. It's tiring! But with every waking hour – as doubts seep in when we're not looking, or we get blindsided from a trusted source – we can't help but feel the guilt and anguish. Have we done enough?

I'm lucky in this regard. I'm not my brother's parent; I'm his sister. And our family adopted Scott, so we haven't had to live out the birth trauma and the guilt that so many families go through with any child either born with or developing a disability. All the stages of grief are experienced – denial, anger, bargaining, depression and acceptance – either in a few days or over 50+ years. Some people get stuck in denial and never get any further; most work through each stage in their own way, until the next hurdle. While it may be to a lesser extent, with each new obstacle we tend to go through it all over again.

Not having lived that initial trauma doesn't mean that we, as Scott's adopted family, don't keenly feel our own inadequacies. Time and again we come across situations of unnecessary heartache for Scott. In fact, I feel a strong sense of obligation, having made the commitment to take Scott into our family, to provide him with a better life. If we fail to do that, it's like we're letting down not only him, but his wonderful foster parents who had him before us, the social workers who entrusted us to him, and everyone who knows us. Have we done enough?

Is there an answer? Only that you could give every waking hour and it would probably still not be enough. But you can do plenty. And everything that you do will have a real impact if you work smart. Ensure you are taking care of yourself, so you can then truly be there for them – however much you can.

So it's the 'working smart' that I can help you with. It's the quality and thoughtfulness of the support you get and give for your family member that can make such a huge difference. You need to employ a dedicated integration aide, quality therapists, a contemporary medical team, and a team of support workers that have not only skill in care, but are interactive in nature.

How do you know if you have a great team or not? Ah, there's the rub!

Throughout this book, I will highlight some of the common issues around quality support for people – particularly those with limited mobility and limited or no speech – and the common sense solutions that we can implement to improve things.

Regardless of the difficulties, barriers, ignorance and struggles, I'm here to tell you that people with disability – all children and adults with any sort of disability, social limitation or learning difficulty – can live an incredibly happy life.

They can be involved in the decision-making for their daily living and future goals – no matter how rudimentary that may be. They can reach their potential if they have the right people to help them to see the possibilities, to have a voice and to be involved in the community. And you – as parents and support workers – can have an incredibly rich, meaningful and joyful relationship with them. I know this because, from both sides of the fence, I've seen it, I've experienced it, I've lived it.

I guess being the eldest of six kids growing up – three of whom had some form of special needs to be addressed – set me up for a lifetime of interest in the field of disability. There's myself, my brother Peter, my step-siblings Lizzie and Robby, then Ben – and we adopted Scott into our family when he was four years old. More about him in a moment.

Briefly, straight out of high school I spent three years working full-time in an institutional special school, and I've been a support worker in homes, caring for children with disability – some for a few visits and others for many years. I've travelled internationally, being the support worker to clients in wheelchairs who use communication boards to get their thoughts across, and have cheered on sporting teams at wheelchair soccer, and balloon football throughout many seasons.

While I now run leadership and teambuilding programs – specialising in creating positive cultures, teaching personality styles and management skills in my business, Mzuri Training – the real impetus for writing this book comes from my experiences working with, supporting and advocating for my brother Scott, now that he lives in a supported accommodation.

For a more detailed biography of my professional and personal experience in teaching, training and being an 'experiential expert' in the field of disabilities, please find the link to 'Julienne's Background Biography' and 'Scott's Background Biography' at <http://www.mzuritraining.com.au/resources.html>.

My mother, Sandra, is an extraordinary woman in many ways. I am the eldest of our brood and when I was 15, in addition to the five children between them, Mum and my then step-father, David, made the decision to adopt my brother Scott, a little boy with extraordinary hurdles to overcome. Mum calls Scotty her 'chosen child'.

It's not just the act of formally adopting a child with significant disabilities, but everything my mum's done in her life that I find quite extraordinary; I feel genuinely honoured to be her daughter.

Scott was the most gorgeous three-and-a-half year old little boy you've ever seen. Beautiful big blue eyes, thick wavy brown hair and a smile that lit up the room. He was an absolute delight – and our whole family loved him to bits. How he came to be with us is a book in and of itself, but let's just say that there was a state-wide appeal to seek new parents for him, with a broadsheet newspaper entitled 'One Last Chance for Scott'. If someone didn't adopt him and take him into their homes, he would be institutionalised for the rest of his life. Long story short, our family was lucky enough to be able to bring him home to us.

Scott has cerebral palsy quadriplegia and is vision-impaired, an epileptic and asthmatic. While he can make sounds, he cannot form words. It must have been excruciatingly tough for him to lose his parents, then his adopted parents, then his foster parents before finally finding a new family, all before turning four years old – especially when he can't walk, talk or see.

Our family took the perspective, given to us by a doctor who pointed out to us that most people with cerebral palsy are not affected intellectually so to 'always give him the benefit of the doubt'. We have tried to hold to this approach his entire life, always giving him the benefit of the doubt.

When she reached her early 50s, my always fit and healthy, yoga instructor mother developed rheumatoid arthritis and knew that she couldn't continue to physically look after Scott, now an adult. So, after an eighteen month difficult process, he was placed in a brand new, purpose-built home to live in with a respected provider.

After my mother and I completed a personal development course, Scott expressed interest in doing it too, and the first few questions were about what goals he had. We had no idea how we were going to work with Scott, but using his yes/no answers like a multiple choice process, he came alive. We started to discover that Scott had deep concerns about his life and health. We were able to pinpoint that he was concerned about his back pain, his finances and the staffing at his house.

Family images

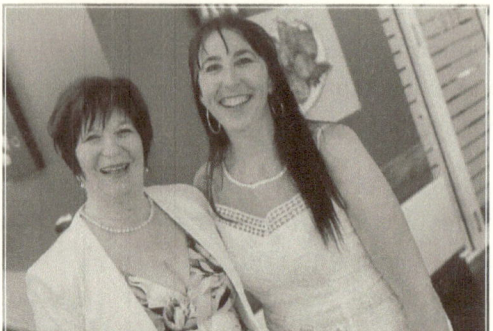

Mum (Sandra) and me at her 70th birthday party, 2016.

Mum (Sandra) with Scott at her 70th birthday party, 2016.

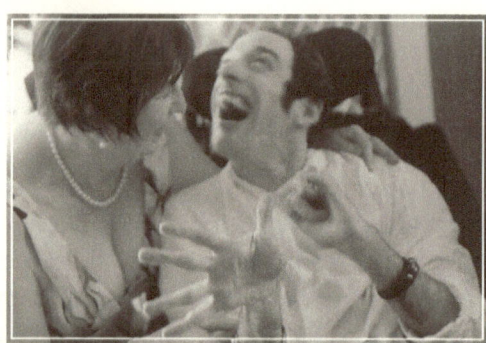

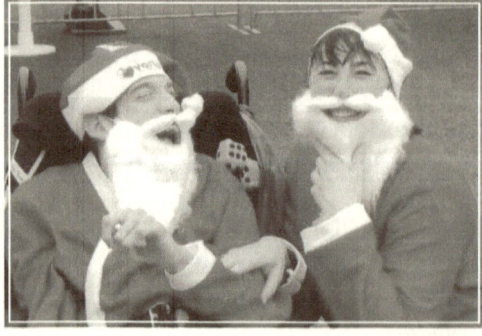

Scott and me doing the Santa Fun Run walk, Melbourne, 2012.

Scott and me relaxing together, 2010.

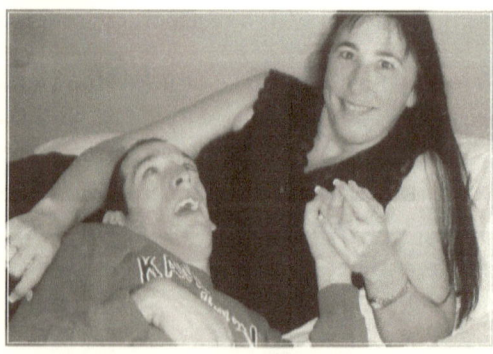

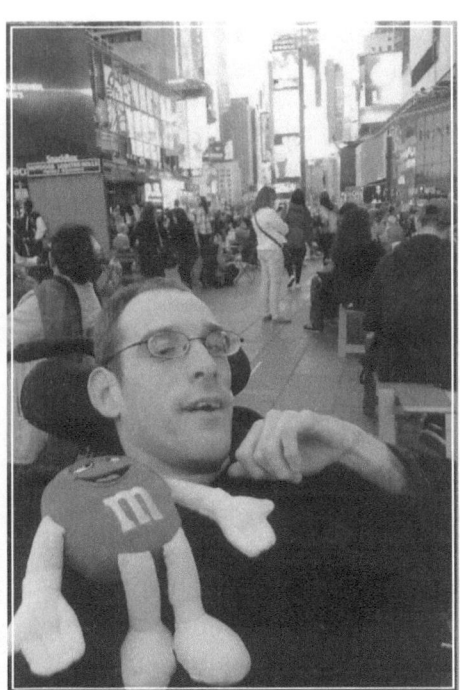

Scott at Times Square in New York City, USA, 2014.

Our immediate family, 2016 – From left: Ben, Scott, Sandra (Mum), Peter and me.

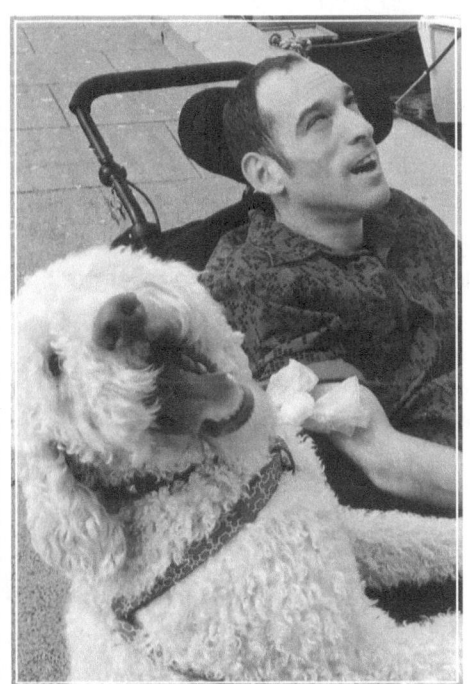

Scott with his dog Jimmy, 2017.

He wanted to travel, to learn, and especially to help other people with disability.

This began a cascade of events, with us spending more time with him to start achieving some of his goals. The more time we spent with him, the more we became concerned that some of the aspects of his care and his equipment – such as his wheelchair – needed urgent improvement.

And so, it wasn't until Scott was in his early 30s that we started having to advocate for him. We had to learn what happens when you speak up and make waves. What works and what doesn't in the complex care system? Which battles do you choose to fight and which ones are better to let go of? And how far do you push? We're still learning.

Since that time, we've achieved getting a special wheelchair designed for him, which significantly reduced his back pain. He's also got a new communication system that's opening up his world of expressing independent thought, and he has his beautiful pet dog Jimmy for company. It really proved to us that with the right support, just about anything is possible. With the help of an extraordinary disability support worker, Rob, Mum and I were able to bring some of Scott's dreams of travel to reality, surviving incredibly long flights, having a blast at Disney World, exploring New York City, completing his personal development course, having fabulous nights out and making fantastic new friends.

Scott has written his thoughts at the beginning of each chapter, as a contributing author. These are his words, painstakingly communicated through various means of discussion, auditory scanning and selecting 'yes' to the various ideas he wanted to express. It's amazing what you can do with time, patience and a solid 'yes' to communicate! He worked with at least three different people, using a communication matrix as well as approving different statements to gauge his responses, then reading back to him what was written in the previous session to confirm if it was correct. 'Are we on the right track? Does it need tweaking? Is it perfect now?' He was amazingly specific. When you read his words, please know that it was no small feat for him to express them to you.

I really want to thank you for picking up this book and reading it. My awesome brother Scott and I hope you get a lot of insights, ideas, inspiration and clarification from it. But ultimately – even though I'm going to highlight some of the nightmares associated with traditional disability care – I want to leave you with a sense of optimism. It can be tough and it can be frustrating, but there is so much good that can be done with just a little tweaking – just a slight recalibration in the way we approach day-to-day support of people with disability. There is joy and possibility and real hope ahead.

Additional Resources

— 'Welcome To Holland' 1987 - poem by Emily Perl-Kingsley Down Syndrome Association. http://www.dsasc.ca/uploads/8/5/3/9/8539131/welcome_to_holland.pdf.

— Video representation of the poem: 'Welcome To Holland' https://www.youtube.com/watch?v=ZMPa2NIAsyE

Chapter 2

Revolution? It's Time!

This chapter is so important. Living at home for most of my life made going into a group home difficult. It's definitely time to make some big changes. Staff have got to be better at their jobs. We need to keep the good ones and get rid of the bad ones.

Scott Clough

With the introduction of the National Disability Insurance Scheme (NDIS), the findings of the Royal Commission into Institutional Responses to Child Abuse, and with self-advocacy happening across the country, I believe it's the right time to instigate a cultural shift in the field of disability. Organisations like Inclusion International are getting worldwide traction, fiercely advocating and putting on quality conferences for those in this field.

No longer is authority the sole discerner of power. With the #MeToo campaign highlighting sexual harassment across the world and the #RealMenDon'tHit campaign addressing domestic violence, we know that speaking up for social change in our community really can work. We've seen with the Australian plebiscite into same sex marriage that people power can make significant change – not just in laws, but more importantly through social acceptability in the eyes of the community.

When it comes to disability, the system has been broken for a long time, and there are some very big things happening around the world to fix it. That's awesome, but let's get real here. The lifestyle of the average person with limited physical and/or intellectual capabilities hasn't really changed very much.

The structural and funding model absolutely had to change – which it's in the throes of doing here in Australia – but I put it to you that it's a cultural change that needs to happen now as well.

A #ridewithme, #marraigeequality type of social uprising to highlight that we stand with and for people with disability, as well as their support workers and families.

To be frank, I don't think the general public have a clue what's been going on behind some closed doors. The community will only insist on change if they know what's been going on, and what they can do change it.

Friedrich Nietzsche, a German philosopher, cultural critic, composer, and poet said: 'People don't want to hear the truth because they don't want their illusions destroyed.'

Are you ready to hear the truth about what's been happening in disability care? Here we go ...

In 2013 the Australian Government established the Royal Commission into Institutional Responses to Child Abuse. The final report from the commission was released on 15 December 2017. The Royal Commission mainly focused on religious groups but also included disability group homes, and the word used to describe the stories they heard was 'shameful'.

There are 300,000 children in Australia with a disability, and it can be said that about 26,700 of them have been, or are being, violently sexually abused.[1] This does not include adults with disability, and it's a conservative estimate.

One of the findings was that children with a disability have a 2.88 times higher risk of being victims to sexual violence than children who do not have a disability.

The likely 'true' prevalence estimate of sexual violence against children with a disability is about 8.9%.[2] This is how we can estimate the probable reality that 26,700 Australian children have been victims of violent sexual assault.

The conclusions of three different studies on abuse were that we need to train staff in institutions to recognise the signs of abuse, to report these signs to their managers and to take action to ensure the child is safe. The studies specifically recommended educational programs to teach the conditions where abuse becomes a higher risk, and how to prevent that occurring.[3]

While I want to let that all sink in for a moment – and to reiterate the data that says serious, violent sexual abuse is a reality for many thousands of Aussie children – I don't want to focus solely on the devastatingly bad. There is so much incredibly awesome work being done by self-advocates, inspiring families, innovative organisations and incredibly dedicated disability support workers, in Australia and around the world.

The majority of people who take care of people with disability, however, are their parents and family members.

— More than 13% of the population are carers, including 217,800 Victorians who are primary carers, assisting with communication, mobility and self-care.

— Nearly 300,000 Victorians with a severe or profound disability (94% needing assistance) are assisted by family members or friends.

— Carers are people of all ages and backgrounds. Most are aged between 35 and 54, but more than 20% of carers are 75 years or older, and the majority (71%) are women.

— About half of all primary carers (56%) are reliant on a government pension, but only 37% have other jobs. Consequently, 47% of primary carers have low incomes.

Here's what I find fascinating: 49% of carers take on a caring role because they believe they can provide better care than any other available services. (And they're probably right.)

In 2015, the annual cost to replace all unpaid carers with support workers was estimated to be $60.3 billion. And while that's a powerful thought, here's the kicker. As today's parent-carers get older and perish, it is anticipated that there will be a major decrease in the number of family carers compared to people needing care, over the next 15–20 years.[4]

Australia joined most of the world by signing and becoming a state party to the United Nations Convention of the Rights of Persons with a Disability (CRPD) in 2007–08. The convention also includes the UK, Europe, Canada, South America, India, China, most of the Middle East and 48 out of the 54 countries in Africa. (The USA has not yet progressed to accession to state party.) The main purpose of this convention – the first human rights treaty of the twenty-first century – is to protect, promote and ensure the full enjoyment of human rights by persons with disability, under the law.

Two of the guiding principles underlying the Convention are:

— Respect for inherent dignity, individual autonomy including the freedom to make one's own choices, and independence of persons

— Full and effective participation and inclusion in society.[5]

So, how is everyone going? Well, in 2013 the UK was struggling, but have made some real changes since.

Dr Jim Elder-Woodward OBE, the Independent Chair of the Scottish Independent Living Coalition, has been spearheading a lot of the good work being done in the UK to address some shortcomings. I think his frustrations were showing when he stated:

> It is the case, for example, that the bright, rosy future depicted by the good intentions behind many pieces of domestic legislation and international conventions quite often play out very dimly in the day-to-day lives of many disabled people …
>
> … I remember being in residential care; being put in a queue to go to the toilet; being forced to eat something I hated; being given help by someone I disliked intensely; and being told when to go to bed. Now, I live in my own home, having retired as a senior social work manager. I decide who should provide the practical support I need. I am also part of the civic and cultural life of my local community. Without the years of campaigning alongside other disabled activists for such a lifestyle, I'd probably still be isolated back in that queue to go to the toilet.[6]

Australia is due to put in an important report to the UN committee in September 2018. Our 'List of Issues' includes 35 areas that we've been specifically told to address. There is a lot of work to be done!

'The future depends on what we do in the present'.

Mahatma Gandhi

With the good work of the United Nations, organisations like Inclusion International running international conferences, popular TV shows now depicting people with disability in thought-provoking roles, and the recent NDIS rollout across Australia, now feels like the right time for a cultural revolution.

For those in our 40s or older, you may recall how drinking and driving used to be something that people just did. People drove home drunk quite often, and just drove on the back roads to avoid getting caught! We all knew it wasn't great, but apathy reigned, and it was an accepted norm.

Then a big media campaign started. The community in Australia was educated about the horrors of drunk driving using graphic TV ads with hard-hitting slogans ('If you drink and drive, you're a bloody idiot'). Moralistic and socially acceptable alternatives were heavily promoted ('designated drivers', night buses, all-night trains, etc.). The focus went from it not being about you, but about the other people you can kill if you drive while drunk.

The result is that while people still do drive while drunk, and police are still out there doing random breath tests, the community attitude and general practice have completely changed. It is now totally uncool to drink and drive, and socially acceptable to say, 'I'm driving so I'm limiting my drinking tonight.' The community in general (and past offenders specifically) have gone from apathy to action. They take keys away from people who have had too much to drink and call them cabs home. They say, 'I'm driving,' and order soft drinks, or pre-organise public transport or taxis home.

I want to help create that same sort of cultural change to introduce specific dialogue and expectations (from apathy to action) in disability care. We need to create a new 'normal' among all who work with and care for people with disability, particularly those with limited mobility and little to no speech. I admit to sometimes feeling like the different providers, practitioners and workers who have assisted my brother of the years are the enemy. Frustration can seem never-ending, and every avenue you explore to get any result leads to longer delays, increased inaction and less responsibility taken for anything. There are times when it really has seemed all too hard and extremely distressing – and I'm just Scott's sister. If I have felt that way, imagine what my mother, and of course Scott himself, must have gone through over the years.

But I also know that huge goals have been achieved, efforts have been made to do the best for Scott by his support network, and a massive amount of love has been ever-present between us as a family.

When in anger or frustration, if an issue is not immediately fixable the distress can be overwhelming. The last thing we want to do – but often the most defusing and ultimately helpful activity – is to see the situation from the perspective of the enemy. What is happening from the support worker/provider/school's position? What are their restrictions and concerns? Sometimes, only after looking at things from this angle can a workable (or at least partial) solution present itself. Solutions are not always fail-safe, or perfect, or consistent, but they are a step forward. There is usually a way through!

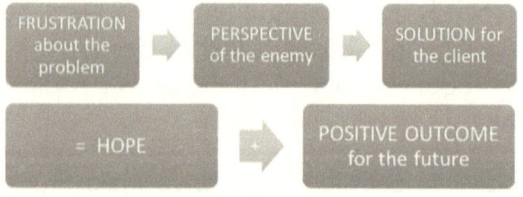

What is required by all support providers is a willingness to listen and pro-actively respond to their clients and family members. When this happens, while frustrations can still arise, solutions can be implemented.

Some people with limited ability do not feel that they are considered a real person. That the concept of personhood, individuality and being self-determinate is something they 'might one day' achieve. Now is that time!

> *'Not being able to speak is not the same as not having anything to say.'*
>
> Anne McDonald

And people with disability have plenty to say!

Chapter 3

Choices, Choices, Choices

It's important to me to have choices about the food I have to eat, and the drinks I drink. I also like to have a say in the clothes I wear, or at least be told what it is that I'm wearing. It still happens that someone puts clothes on me that belong to the other guys who live in my house, which makes me frustrated and angry as it feels disrespectful. I don't get to choose how often I get to see family; I rarely get asked about pain relief, or just if I want more drink. I'm always thirsty!

I'm taken shopping often, but choices are made for me, and I don't get to confirm those choices. I really enjoy shopping for things for myself, or gifts for others, but I don't like it when my mum and sister stop at a dress shop. They can take ages and I get annoyed!

But it's the big things I don't get a choice with; who I live with and who cleans and showers me. When I have to put up with someone I don't like or trust caring for me, I feel frustrated and upset. But, I'm the happy smiling guy! (Laughs)

I'm smiley on the outside but still scared and frustrated on the inside.

I can say 'yes' – I just want to be asked.

Scott Clough

As the 'Get Real' girl, if something's not working, I like to declare that and make small, immediate changes for the short term while beginning the process for more significant changes long term. Being proactive is an essential part of being an Interactive Care worker.

Interactive Care is made up of eight themes. The first theme to Interactive Care is 'Choices, Choices, Choices (People are not pot plants!)'.

For most of us, making choices is an everyday occurrence that we take for granted. But for many people with disability, having any real say in their lives can be a rarity. The art of making choices is different and sometimes difficult depending on the disability that the person has. Nevertheless, to make a choice is a self-determining exercise. To choose demonstrates individuality and power over one's own life.

To decide is to be self-determinate. It's the difference between being alive and having a life – to be able to make major life choices like where you live, what you do each day and which medication you are on. The ability to make both major choices and little everyday choices (what I want to eat today, where I want to go today, how I want to get there, which staff member I want to work with me) is a fundamental human right.

I know of several group homes where a client's choice of clothing, food, drink, TV shows, outings and activities is only occasionally given.

Sometimes my passion about this can get overwhelming for my brother Scott. As my mother Sandra, our disability support worker Rob and I set off with Scott on our trip to America, I was all about him being able to choose everything for his trip. What do you want for breakfast? How do you want your eggs? How many pieces of toast? Do you want to look at the planes? Do you need to go to the toilet?

I remember we were only halfway to the States and Scotty wasn't responding very clearly to me, and then stopped responding at all. I became concerned, asking if there was something wrong. Had we forgotten something? Is everything okay?

Rob, bless him, intuitively cottoned on and just asked him: 'Scott, are there too many choices?'

Scott's eyes brightened, and he slammed his hand down. 'Yes!'

I was bombarding him with something he so rarely gets to do; it was too much for him. I was drowning him in choices! I apologised and we all had a bit of a laugh about it. I backed off with the choices for a while, but over the next day or two, he got quicker and more decisive about what he wanted, and within three days he was making all his own choices, all day.

The problem, of course, is often not one of capacity or ability to choose. It's that for busy support workers and family carers – often looking after several people at a time – giving all clients choice takes time, effort, money, ingenuity and creativity. The weekly food shopping, for example, is often at best a group menu decision, or there's no input from the clients at all. And even if they have all decided 10 days earlier that they want a roast this Sunday, there's usually little chance of altering that if one person wants something different on the day. I acknowledge and applaud those supported accommodation places where clients do have the choice of their meals and drinks – and when and where they have them.

I also appreciate that there is a need to balance choice with quality and practicality. I guess there are some clients who would subsist on soft drink and chocolate if we let them! But in my experience, it's usually the opposite. Scott's favourite thing is to go out for lunches and dinners because he loves good food. He usually orders a steak, or prawns, or yummy Indian food – but even then, choice can be limited by budget, time and dietary requirements!

As family members, we tend to hold on to the things we know; without realising it, we can actually restrict our people with disability's choices. When my mother was out to lunch with Scott last year, his new disability support worker ordered Scott a salad. Mum reacted, 'Oh he won't eat that!'

The support worker, to his credit, retorted, 'Yes he will!' And he did! He loved it! Mum would never have thought that he'd choose a salad. So our own beliefs can be limiting and we need to encourage everyone to try new things!

What does a lifetime of not being offered choice – about virtually anything in their lives – do to people? If someone never has a say in what they eat each night, how on earth would they feel empowered to make choices about the big things in their life? Their self-worth, self-determinism, willingness to try anything new, or confidence to fight for the important things can all be affected.

Of course, allowing choice makes things more difficult to co-ordinate. It's much easier for the provider if everyone just accepts what's offered to them. The budgets get adhered to, the house gets cleaned and everyone is happy. (Except the people being supported.)

Once last thing about choice. We currently house many people with disability together in state institutions or community housing, and I don't think this is always the best decision. It's done so that accommodation can be supported, transport organised, activities done – it's all very practical. But does it actually achieve the end goal of a quality life for the people we're meant to be supporting?

When discussing writing this book with my friend Marlena, she told me that one thing that really annoys her is so many people talking about 'inclusion' while placing people with disability all together in one place. We shouldn't ignore some of the excellent support that is already in our society and take advantage of being in the community whenever possible. This will now hopefully be a more possible reality with the NDIS.

Housing people separately from their families, and living with other people with disability, can sometimes lose the most important thing – and the one thing the NDIS is supposed to create more of: choice!

Campbell Brown, who has significant physical disabilities and slurred speech, summarised this issue very bluntly to my mum one day. He was able to articulate that, 'I had to go to school with all these f*ck-heads, and now I have to live with them too!'

The extension of this concept is that provocative tagline: people are not pot plants! We feed and water plants; we clean the leaves and make them shiny. We clear the pot of weeds, and even re-pot them as they grow. We like them, so we might say nice things to them and ensure they get some sun. But that's about it.

Pot plants don't talk back to us. They don't say, 'I want to go here. I want this. I don't want that.' They also don't have annoying family members making complaints, asking for extras and questioning your policies!

I'm afraid this really is how we sometimes care for people, particularly if they have limited mobility, and limited or no speech. We feed and water them and give them something to do during the day (no matter how trivial it might be). We put clothes on them and we say nice things to them – because that's our job. When they're happy people and they behave well, they're easy to look after.

Those people who display difficult behaviours are not so easy to like. You see, pot plants are not supposed to speak up, talk back to us or be difficult. They're not supposed to cause trouble. For those with intellectual or social conditions that limit understanding or communication, the life of a pot plant can be a metaphor for how they live their life – unless we break out of that mindset.

Of course, we don't think we believe these things, but our actions reveal the truth. We can expect a lot from them! They have so much to give, to contribute, to say! Those with extremely limited capacity can still feel, and love, and be. Whenever there's an opportunity for them to choose, we need to interact with them and see if we can make those choices a reality. I call this 'Empathy, not Apathy'. We need to accept their limitations, but not ours or our organisations.

But, I hear some of you say, what if they make really inconvenient choices? Yep, they just might. As their supporter, find out the reason for the odd or problematic choice. You can bargain with them, negotiate terms! Every request can at least be heard and acknowledged, and an attempt made to accommodate for them. Explain why they can't do something if it's not possible.

When Scott was about eight years old, he was very agile. He couldn't walk or even crawl properly, but he could definitely get around! We often put him on the lounge room floor and he would get himself across the room, out the sliding door, onto the large rug on our patio, down the long wooden ramp built for the wheelchair by my step-father, and onto our rough gravel driveway. Sometimes he was so quick, we wouldn't realise until he was covered in gravel and eating dirt!

My mum was concerned that he would hurt himself if we weren't vigilant in stopping him. One day, while relaying his latest escapade to her friend Campbell Brown, he just gave her a knowing cheeky smile and said, 'He'll learn. He'll toughen up!'

One last point on the theme of choices, and the way providers tend to approach this. Promoted everywhere on websites are most organisations' core values and commitments to their clients' right to choose. That's great – but the reality it's sometimes quite different.

One example involves the right to choose your own doctor. Say an older lady in a group home with learning and physical disabilities, but with speech, has clearly expressed a desire to change her general practitioner. She doesn't like the way he talks to her disability support worker rather than her. She doesn't like his gruff answers to her requests and she doesn't think he listens to her concerns. She's been very vocal to the house staff about seeing a different doctor, but the reply is standard. Everyone in her home goes to that doctor, and they all go together, so she has to go too, and that won't change.

As an Interactive Carer (either as a family member or paid worker), one of your roles is to help people with disability find and express their thoughts and preferences. It's all about living in a deliberate, self-determinate way. To have choice is to not just be alive, but to have a life.

Each theme of Interactive Care has been born from dissatisfaction, and being compelled to disrupt the traditional disability 'care' system. Therefore, it tends to start with a frustration and examples of *why*. We need to address and be mindful of these issues. But many of you may have heard about the typical boss who tells you not to bother coming to them with a problem unless you've also got a solution? Well, similarly I feel it's important, as family members, when having concerns about the standard of care your person with disability is receiving, we need to bear in mind this personal policy:

> If you've not prepared to be part of the solution, you forfeit your right to complain.

Sounds great when directing this towards your staff, or even your kids, but it's sometimes quite a difficult thing to accomplish when you're advocating for someone who needs your voice, and others are being paid to supposedly do the right thing.

But this truly is one of the keys to the way forward. I've often been livid at something I think is simply common sense that hasn't been done for Scott – and I just want to scream, 'Think about it!' at whomever got distracted with 100 other things and missed the one thing I've noticed straight away. Point it out, sure, but if it requires something to assist the supporting people to be able to do it properly next time, it's our job as the complainer to offer to be part of the solution.

If I notice that, six weeks after being told about needing to replace his shoes, they are still not replaced, then I'll take Scott out to get new ones. It gives us a chance to spend time together and I know I'll get the right ones. If I'm concerned that Scott's dog Jimmy isn't being fed the right amount of food, or his water bowl isn't being cleaned, rather than complain about it, I'll make a poster for all support workers to easily follow, so they all know what to do.

We were lucky enough to get to work with a wonderful speech therapist who started Scott on a new communication method recently. Even though she made a video and a handout to give to all staff, instead of just emailing it off to them and hoping it would get to everyone smoothly, I made sure I attended their staff meetings to show them all personally. It takes time and effort, but it's not useful to just get furious at every shortcoming you experience with any provider.

If you're not prepared to be part of the solution, you forfeit your right to complain. So, in the spirit of giving some solutions, without any assumption of your current situation, at the end of each chapter I will offer some action steps that we can all do if you have a concern befitting any of the themes being explored.

Strategy Solutions

A. What can you as a family member do?

— Displaying what sort of choices your person with disability likes to make is a great way to encourage support workers to give them choice. A colourful tray display if they use a wheelchair, the front page of a daily diary, a laminated sign, or a poster in their room or on the fridge are good places to put it.

— Modelling how they choose, and what things they like to have a choice about, is a great way to connect with and model their abilities to support workers.

B. What can support workers and their providers do?

— I put it to you that it's our job, as support workers, to find time every shift to do different things with each person. Read, play games, try art, enjoy a show, sing and dance – one thing involving them, when you've finished showering them, or giving them dinner, or cleaning the kitchen or doing the washing.

— It's your job to do more than look after them, like pot plants, but to interact with them about things that they're interested in. It's the difference between, say, putting them in front of the TV to watch a program, and sitting down and chatting to them about the program as it progresses. Football, for example, is so much more fun to watch when everyone cheers or moans when your side gets a goal. It's a bit of a soulless experience when everyone else is busy doing other things while you watch it on your own. It's not just choice, but interaction and support with that choice that is the interactive difference.

C. What can we do as a movement, (with and for people with disability)?

— If you are a self-advocate, I'm here to tell you, you have the right to decide. 'I decide' is your new mantra. You might have to negotiate with people; you might need to save up your money or change your routine to earn what you want. There might be delays, and you might even make a mistake or two. You might become unpopular, but the more people with disability who self-advocate, the easier and more acceptable it will become to exercise your right to choose.

Additional Resources

— Tedx Talks 2015, 'The Art of Dreaming | Maithri Goonetilleke', *YouTube*, <https://www.youtube.com/watch?v=7bGS6xaX7m4>.

Chapter 4

Horrors and Heroes

My frustration boils up and over when I think of what so many people like me have been through. Something has to improve! I know others who have been mistreated or neglected. It breaks my heart to not be able to help them. I've encountered impatient staff members, terrible taxi drivers, or just people who say mean things, thinking I don't understand and knowing I can't do anything to stop them.

Just you wait! (Cheeky smile)

But I'm so grateful for the heroes I know. Those who advocate for me. I can get embarrassed when my sister or mother are making a scene, trying to improve something for me, but I'm also very grateful. They express things better and louder than I can.

I want to say that I know what it is to be abused and neglected. I've experienced it first-hand. Those times stay with you forever.

My heroes are:

— *My mum, Sandra: She took me in when no one else would. She calls me her 'chosen child' and she loves me.*

— *Norma and Lyndsay: They kept me alive and gave me a life, with love and fun.*

— *Damien and Pauline: my main carers when I was young.*

> — *Rob: my awesome support worker and mate. He's so funny (he makes me laugh all the time) and gentle and he just 'gets' me.*
>
> — *Lyndon and other practitioners like Sam and Anne: their intuition and skill make my day.*
>
> — *My sister, Julienne: for the time she spends with me and the passion she has to make things better.*
>
> — *My current group of awesome disability support workers, particularly Olivia.*
>
> — *All the people throughout my life who have been kind, fun and advocated for me when I really needed it.*

Scott Clough

Most people don't know the true history of disability care, and what people with disability have had to endure. If you don't know the extent of what has happened, how can you understand where they are coming from?

I will also balance this with what some amazing organisations are doing and extraordinary accomplishments from different people.

This Interactive Care theme is: 'The Horrors and The Heroes; You need to understand the past to comprehend the fight for a better future.'

So, it's time for a history lesson.

People with a difference have been treated poorly throughout history. Children and adults with any sort of disability were:

- killed, drowned, burnt or abandoned in ancient times all over the world

- housed in the basements of prisons in America in the early 1600s

- dehumanised in orphanages and asylums across Europe in the 1800s

- found handcuffed to their beds in an 'Institution for Idiots' in America in the late 1800s[7]

— subjected to propaganda in 1939, when Adolf Hitler stated that it 'was the best time for the elimination of the incurably ill' and authorised people with disability to be neglected until they died of starvation or disease.

From the early 1900s, disability was viewed through an 'incurable' medical lens, so people – particularly those with any intellectual disability – were put away 'out of sight and out of mind' in institutions (Llewellyn et al., 2016). They were considered 'patients' and were 'put away' in large-scale establishments with nurses and hospital beds.

Accounts of every form of degradation have been published. Inhumane punishments for certain behaviours, cruel therapies, rape, torture and extreme neglect. The emotional damage was no doubt beyond any of our comprehension.

'Forgotten Australians' is the term used by the Australian Senate to describe children who were brought up in orphanages, children's homes, institutions or foster care in Australia between 1920 and the 1970s.

Approximately 500,000 children were placed in institutional care at this time, many of whom experienced neglect and abuse. In 2009, the Australian Government formally apologised to Forgotten Australians and child migrants on behalf of the nation.[8]

Here in Australia, in the mid-1970s, a woman started working at St Nicholas Hospital in Melbourne, when she met a young girl with cerebral palsy.

> When I first met Anne, she was 12 years old, the height of a 4-year-old but skeletally thin, writhing on the floor at St. Nicholas Hospital, a state institution for children believed to be profoundly mentally retarded. 'Who's that?' 'That's McDonald. She'll be dead in 6 months. We can't feed her'.
>
> No therapy, no education, no wheelchair, no toys, no clothes of your own and not enough to eat or drink – just the floor and a cot. It wasn't much of a life, but Anne enjoyed whatever there was to enjoy. She still had her trademark grin and wicked sense of humour. This probably saved her life, because it led me to choose her for a communication project when she was 16 and weighed under 13 kilos.[9]

Rosemary taught Anne how to spell and communicate; Anne then asked to leave the institution. Court cases, media reports and general condemnation from the establishment followed, but Anne prevailed and won her case. She lived with Rosemary and her partner for the rest of her life, achieving a university degree (using many different communication assistants) and co-writing the book *Annie's Coming Out*, which was later made into a film.

Rosemary Crossley continues to be a controversial figure today, teaching people to communicate by methods which include the physical assistance of another person. She works tirelessly (without any funding) to help anyone who wants her assistance. Her tenacity, creativity and life's work is internationally recognised – while still discredited by others. I believe she will go down in history as one of the true heroes of our time.

No doubt we must protect people with disability from manipulation, misrepresentation and abuse of funds. My position is that we must judge every case on its merits, and in order to do this we have to acknowledge any technique that can be proven to work, by multiple people being able to get the same results. Otherwise, we could be using our own judgements to severely limit others.

> *'If you judge a fish by its ability to climb a tree, it will live its whole life believing that it is stupid.'*
>
> *Albert Einstein*

Societal changes started to occur in Australia during the late 60s and early 70s, with the Handicapped Child's Allowance in 1974 encouraging parents to care for their disabled children at home. Public awareness also increased with the International Year of Disabled Persons in 1981. The National Disability Strategy 2010–2020 has paved the way for other reforms, the signing of the United Nations Charter for People with Disabilities, and the complete change in Australia's funding process for people with disability with the new National Disability Insurance Scheme (NDIS).

As a society, we have definitely moved on from the old medical model, into what's called the social model.[10] This was developed by activists who started the 'independent living movement'; from the person with disability's point of view this says: 'Here we are. We are part of society, and the only real limitation we have is from you as a society not making things accessible to us.'

Most people with disability don't need nurses; they are not sick. They just need assistance to do everyday things.

Yes, we've come a long way – in many ways. Yet, for some people, not a whole lot has changed.

The Australian Bureau of Statistics (ABS) released summary findings in 2012 of a survey of disability, ageing and carers. It showed that violence against people with disability in institutional and residential settings is 'Australia's hidden shame'.

The evidence of this national epidemic 'is extensive and compelling, and this blight on our society and can no longer remain ignored and unaddressed'.[11]

The number of people with disability who are being drugged as a way of managing behaviours of concern is frightening. It's a practise known as 'chemical restraint', and in May 2017, the ABC (Australia) reported that 99% of people with an intellectual disability, and living in a group home, were on psychotropic drugs – but only 46% actually had a mental illness.

The Australian Government produced a document titled 'Understanding safeguarding practices for children with disability when engaging with organisations' in 2017. In it they state that 'Children with disability have a nearly four times higher risk of experiencing violence than their non-disabled peers.'[12]

So serious abuse really is happening, right here, right now. What are the risk factors for this abuse, and why is it still occurring?

In 2011 the World Health Organization (WHO), after reviewing existing different studies, concluded that the following were risk factors:

— segregated settings;

— children with disability being alone with an adult;

— closed and locked settings;

— organisational culture and attitudes such as those supporting a culture of closed communication; and

— poor leadership and organisational governance.[13]

A young man with cerebral palsy was thought to have suffered abuse in January this year (2018). After raising concerns, which were largely ignored by the hospital, his family did something that is illegal in aged care and group homes – they hid a camera in his room. What resulted was clear footage of the physically abusive behaviour by the male nurse.

Who is going to be brave enough to be the first service provider to have mandatory motion detector video cameras (CCTV) in every room, monitored on a regular basis?

As support workers, we must be vigilant, speak up for our clients and keep talking about these issues.

For a much more detailed report – siting additional evidence, reports and statistics to verify all I've said here – download my 'Horrors in Detail' report from the following link:

— 'Interactive Care – Resources', Mzuri Training, <http://www.mzuritraining.com.au/resources.html>

Just as it's vital to be informed about the darker side of the disability field, it's also important to highlight the brilliant, innovative, courageous and outstanding things being achieved for and by people with various disabilities, in Australia and throughout the world. A fraction of the amazing, dedicated, inspiring acts of kindness, passion, skill and courage are celebrated here.

In no particular order – and from my limited perspective – here are some of the heroes in today's disability field:

Support Groups

To all of the wonderful, active support groups for all of the different conditions, disabilities and challenging stories out there. You are heroes to each and every person you spend time with and give guidance, companionship and support to.

Self-advocates

At the 'Having a Say' conference run by VALID in January this year, Miranda Bruyniks, then Deputy Disability Commissioner, was on stage with a wonderful self-advocate; they explained how they had just attended the largest conference on disability in the world. Out of 1000 delegates attending this conference, only three of them actually had a disability! It's time to be including the right people at these events. So self-advocates, we need you! Speak up for yourselves and attend these conferences – 'Nothing about us without us!'

Advocacy Groups

— Inclusion International is the global network of people with intellectual disabilities, with 200 member federations throughout the world. Over the past 50 years, Inclusion International has worked closely with the United Nations, UNESCO, UNICEF, the World Bank and the World Health Organization. They help people with intellectual disabilities to live in the community, to have meaningful contact with their families, to have access to inclusive education and to help advocate in any legal capacity possible. They also have the ear of the United Nations. It doesn't get much higher than that! <http://inclusion-international.org>

— The Victorian Advocacy League for Individuals with Disability (VALID) represents adults with an intellectual disability and their families. VALID is run by and for people with disability and family members, and has particular expertise in networking and providing information to people across Victoria. <https://www.valid.org.au>

— Communication Rights Australia provides specialist information and advocates for people with disability whose human rights have been infringed, giving priority to those with little or no speech. <https://www.caus.com.au>

— Inclusion Australia (NCID) bring together people with intellectual disability and those who are committed to the shared vision of inclusion in all aspects of Australian life. <https://www.inclusionaustralia.org.au>

— Disability Advocacy Network Australia (DANA) is a network of organisations throughout Australia that undertake or provide individual, legal or family advocacy.
<http://www.dana.org.au>

Angels in Disguise

These people are doing amazing things for people with disability.

Stephen Davies

Inventor Stephen Davies is creating prosthetic arms for children in his shed – for free! He was born without a left lower arm and stigmatised as a child for his prosthetic. Now his business Team UnLimbited creates customised 'cool' limbs for children in Wales, UK, and is helping scores of children by making state-of-the-art Spider-Man and Harry Potter-themed prosthetic arms for children all over the world.[14]

Sarah Barton

An Aussie film maker who has produced the film *Defiant Lives*, which documents some of the profound achievements achieved over the past decades in Australia in the disability field. Sarah speaks at conferences, and her film is still shown at presentations around the country.[15]

Rosemary Crossley

The Anne McDonald Centre provides assessment and therapy for people – any age, any diagnosis – with little or no functional speech, providing augmentation communication aids that they can use.[16]

People with Disability rocking the world

Robert Martin

Born with an intellectual disability, New Zealander Robert Martin was abandoned by his parents and institutionalised as a toddler. He now campaigns to ensure others don't endure the same inhumane treatment.

His story has been told in the fascinating book *Becoming a Person*, and Robert was one of Inclusion International's representatives during the negotiations of the CRPD. He then became the first person with an intellectual disability to be elected onto the United Nations Committee which oversees the Convention on the Rights of Persons with Disabilities (CRPD). A tireless worker for change, he is a hero in the disability world.

Marlena Ketene

A totally awesome, world-travelling entertainment journalist, business owner and author. Marlena has a degree in journalism and has interviewed many entertainment celebrities, like Craig David, Snoop Dogg, John Butler, Jessica Irwin, David Copperfield and Russell Brand. She's danced on stage with Pharrell Williams and her hobbies include base jumping, sky-diving and surfing. Marlena travels the world with her flatmate and best mate, Bert, who works as a disability support worker in his day job.

Marlena also happens to have cerebral palsy quadriplegia. She cannot walk or talk and she communicates using a board on her tray. She's never been in the 'system'; she's always lived with her mother or in her own apartment. She relies on support workers – whom she insists on choosing herself – and Bert supports her whenever they go on their overseas trips.

My favourite interview by her – one of her first – is with Russell Brand. I think it's hilarious.[17]

John Cronin

John's Crazy Socks is a father and son venture, inspired by John, a young man with Down syndrome, and his love of colourful and fun socks. They offer over 1200 different socks, and 5% of every pair sold is donated towards the Special Olympics.

Mark Cronin, John's dad, heads a website development company, and together they created this very successful and growing business. His socks are really cool too![18]

As another hero in this chapter, it's great to see that the office of the Disability Services Commissioner has, as of 16 August 2017, been given new powers. They can now make enquiries into any death of a person with disability receiving disability services, send investigators to a service provider during an investigation, or instigate their own investigations into abuse or neglect in the provision of disability services.

Strategy Solutions

A. What can you as a family member do?

— Be vigilant. Get to know the support workers, activity coordinators and other practitioners. Be approachable.

— Drop in occasionally, unannounced, to day centres, schools and group homes – particularly around meal times, so you can see how things operate on a regular basis.

— Be prepared for an emergency. Create a laminated emergency card – so any brand new support worker, nurse in a hospital or ambulance officer can know at a glance how they communicate, eat/drink, show pain, and any additional health concerns (like asthma, epilepsy, allergies or phobias).

— Look up one new support group, disability hero or resource every week. Every Monday night can be Research Night. You'll be amazed what you find. Start with the Resource page on the Mzuri Training website.

B. What can support workers and their providers do?

— The Disability Services Commissioner stated that 22% of complaints made about allegations of physical and sexual assault were made by support workers.

— That is, people seeing something wrong and making a complaint about it. But there's a catch:

> All of these support workers chose to remain anonymous or confidential while making their complaint, which suggests a fear of speaking up and a fear of repercussions from their employer, the service provider.[19]

— If you are a manager in a service provider: what are you doing to provide protection for your staff, and encouragement to report abuse and neglect to you?

— As a support worker there is always someone you can go to if you suspect any form of abuse or neglect. You do not have to have proof, or know who did it – you just need to have a reasonable suspicion or concern. If you don't feel comfortable going to someone within your own organisation, go to elsewhere and please – please tell the family. Sometime they are the only ones who can truly console their person and know what needs to be done.

C. What can we do, as a movement, with and for people with disability?

— If you, as a person with disability, have been, are being, or are concerned about being abused – tell someone! Tell everyone until someone listens. You have the right to be safe.

— As a community we need to no longer say, 'Oh – What a shame!' or, 'How terrible!' when we hear of yet another abuse case come to light. There needs to be outrage and questions asked about legal consequences for perpetrators, and counselling and utmost care taken to help the victim recover and heal. Most importantly it must be stopped and everyone involved made safe – immediately.

Additional Resources

— Baker, R & McKenzie, N 2015, 'Disabled were abused in house of horrors and governments covered it up' <https://www.theage.com.au/national/victoria/disabled-were-abused-in-house-of-horrors-and-governments-covered-it-up-20150408-1mgq13.html>.

— 'FACT SHEET: 6 organisations doing awesome things for people with disability', <http://www.mzuritraining.com.au/resources.html>

— A 30-minute documentary of Robert Martin's journey to become the first intellectually disabled person to be elected onto the UN committee that oversees the Convention on the Rights of Persons with Disabilities: Attitude 2016, 'Robert Martin Makes History', YouTube, <https://www.youtube.com/watch?v=3Mrt9G9kgJA>.

— 4. ABC TV, Four Corners 2014, 'In Our Care', ABC TV, <http://www.abc.net.au/4corners/stories/2014/11/24/4132812.htm>.

— Branley, A 2017, 'Family's battle for justice for daughter who sustained unexplained black eyes, cuts in care', ABC News, <http://www.abc.net.au/news/2017-04-06/familys-battle-for-justice-for-daughter-assaulted-in-care/8402140>.

— Waas, M 1994, 'Bleak House', Los Angeles Times, <http://articles.latimes.com/1994-04-03/magazine/tm-41569_1_forest-haven-bleak-house-institutional-abuse>.

— 'The Murder Of The Handicapped', United States Holocaust Memorial Museum, <https://www.ushmm.org/outreach/en/article.php?ModuleId=10007683>.

— Bawden, A & Campbell, D 2012, 'NHS accused over deaths of disabled patients', The Guardian, <https://www.theguardian.com/society/2012/jan/02/nhs-accused-disabled-patient-deaths>.

— Harkin, L AM 2018, 'Statement regarding the abuse of people with a disability', Disability Services Commissioner, <http://www.oDisability Services Commissioner.vic.gov.au/2018/02/02/statement-regarding-abuse-people-disability/>.

— The Australian Cross Disability Alliance 2015, 'Submission Senate Community Affairs References Committee: 'Inquiry into Violence, Abuse and Neglect against People with Disability in Institutional and Residential Settings' 2015, Australian Cross Disability Alliance, <https://www.aph.gov.au/DocumentStore.ashx?id=3ec383d3-7f51-4029-b9f6-8c6718d4cf31&subId=401199>.

— 'Disability Statistics', Australian Network on Disability, <https://www.and.org.au/pages/disability-statistics.html>.

— UN Guidelines: How To Write and Report about People With Disabilities, 2013, <https://rtcil.drupal.ku.edu/sites/rtcil.drupal.ku.edu/files/images/galleries/Guidelines%208th%20edition.pdf>.

Chapter 5

Embody Leadership Everyday

I feel like giving up when people let me down.

I rely on staff to do all the important things, like to give me food and drink, to help me to sit up, to go to the toilet and to go outside. But also to do fun things, to organise holidays and to speak up when other staff members – like some casuals – are not good enough.

When you do everything for me (or when you don't speak up for me) it makes a huge difference in my world.

Scott Clough

A vital theme for all those supporting people with disability is 'Leadership Regardless of Your Title' (It's your job to advocate for those in your care)'.

Many professionals are now being trained in this concept of leadership – that no matter what your job description entails, no matter what the title on your office door says, you need to show leadership!

This doesn't always feel like the case, however, if we show initiative and are stifled by routine, policy, culture, poor management or, in some organisations, fear of retribution for rocking the boat! Yep – show leadership, stick your neck out, and get it chopped off for your trouble! 'I don't think so …' I hear many of you say.

Well, the ideology behind embodying everyday leadership is that the days of command and control in management are long gone. We have a lot more opportunity to show leadership, create momentum, and make many small, but significant changes – to improve your own job satisfaction, create more team harmony, and to advance the quality of care and inclusion for people with any sort of disability, illness, condition or at-need status.

We are powerful humans, and our attitudes affect those around us.

We all know there are people without any authority who, for better or worse, are the true leaders in any environment. The receptionist who 'runs the place', the disability support worker everyone takes heed of, or the big family dog who dictates the entire family's routine! It's often not the one with the title who holds the cards when it comes to the culture of the place.

> *'Culture eats strategy for breakfast!'*
>
> *Peter Drucker*

Many companies have glossy mission statements on their websites, but the day-to-day reality of the place is often quite different. A poor workplace culture will undermine the slogan on any brochure. A negative, frustrated or apathetic culture ignoring company policy is one possible result, though in disability care I often find the opposite: support workers and managers going above and beyond, working incredibly hard to do the right thing by their clients. Sometimes they do this despite difficult policies, a lack of support and a distinct lack of reward for work undertaken.

A truly positive culture is when the mindset and practice in reality matches the rhetoric on the website, and everyone actively works towards the organisation's (or family's) vision.

As a front-line disability support worker you may not have much authority, but you do have power. You really do. Leading, regardless of title, starts with a sense of your own ability to influence based on what you know to be the right and best thing to do. It's all a question of mindset, confidence and experience.

You see, what sets the great leaders apart from others isn't their higher intelligence, charismatic charm, innovative outlook or any other qualities often attributed to leadership. It lies in their humanity and being able to back themselves: as authentic, purposeful, trustworthy and courageous in their own way. That's how people lead, and that's what others feel compelled to follow and support.

Okay, enough of the conceptual and theoretical. It's time for the practical! Three ways to be a leader in your workplace, regardless of your title:

1. Be friendly – and get to know your people (staff, clients, families).

2. Be generous – with your attention on others.

3. Be brave – and inspire others to be brave.

To delve into this topic more, download my 'Disability Leadership Regardless of Title' PDF at <www.MzuriTraining.com.au/InteractiveCare/Resources>.

Tell me, if you are a disability support worker, teacher, professional carer, council worker in homes, a centre manager or a volunteer – who do you work for? Who is it really? It is the provider, the school, the NDIS, the Government, or the family who requested you? Stop and think about this – and say an answer out loud before reading on. (I'll give you a hint: it's not necessarily those who pay you!)

You work for your client/s. Sorry to providers, city councils, aged care centres, and parents who pay privately for assistance for their people with disability. You may pay them, manage them, discipline them and be responsible for them – but they are not there to serve you.

Being an experienced teacher in several countries, I understand that we are considered mandatory reporters. Regardless of the school we work in, we are duty-bound to look out for the students we teach. Ultimately, they are our clients. I feel it's the same for those supporting people with disability. They are your clients.

Let's say you're hiring new support workers for your family member, or organisation, or yourself. You meet Jenny, who has her Cert IV in Disability and shows a real interest in people with disability. Plus, she has some experience, and says she can handle the job.

At the interview, Jenny appears friendly and confident. When you talk to her about the job, she tells you she's so excited to start. She'll do the active duties and she'll be interactive with the people involved. She'll be on time and continue to be happy and keen to try new things. But there's one thing she wants you to know, up-front – one thing she's not comfortable doing. If she sees someone doing anything suspicious, or intuitively suspects that a client is being hurt or abused in some way, she won't be doing anything about it.

Jenny won't feel comfortable raising any flags, mentioning it to anyone or doing anything practical to protect that person. Okay?

So, are we all good with that? Are we hiring Jenny? Of course not. Put it like that and it sounds ridiculous. Yet, by virtue of the very statistics that have been released, most support workers are either not noticing any abuse or not reporting it. Either way, it's not good enough. All staff – including cooks, cleaners, groundsmen, maintenance staff, managers, OTs, physios, swimming instructors, taxi drivers, visiting nurses, doctors and family visitors – must speak up if something is not right.

As disability support workers, it's your job to advocate for those in your care. It doesn't matter whether you're a casual worker, full time caregiver, a once-off volunteer, or lifetime family member. You do need to use wisdom, of course. Which battles do I choose to fight, and how far do I take this? But when it really matters, you have to be prepared to stand strong and face it.

Late last year, a disturbing story hit the nightly news of a disabled man living in a group home who was sent to hospital, and 'died' in the presence of physicians three times before eventually recovering from his condition. He had become seriously ill from being on a drug cocktail so toxic that his body had no hope of processing it, resulting in his gallbladder turning fully gangrenous.

Even if each drug was legitimately prescribed and administered, as claimed by the provider, where was the observance of this man's health by those paid to look after him? Every time this man was incoherent or in pain, where was the support worker informing someone that something wasn't right? There are many disturbing aspects to this story, including the failure of staff to show any leadership for their client.

Your gut feeling, your intuition, your knowingness is very powerful and usually spot on. These are when you need to act – and take a stand. You all have opportunities to have an impact on a person's life – to make a difference, and to create great connections – just by being you, really listening to them, and taking action! This is leadership.

Here's a basic list of some of the commonly regarded essentials to leading a team:

1. Model the way! Be the change you want to see in the world
    4. A vision for the organisation, and your specific team
    5. Clear, real and honoured core values
    6. Being up-to-date and preparing for changes
    7. Clear and transparent communication that's optimistic in nature
    8. A healthy reward and recognition program for deserving staff

We do not inspire others by showing them how amazing we are, but by being big and loud. Sometime this is what's required, but it's not the end goal. We inspire people by showing them how amazing they are.

'Treat employees like they make a difference, and they will.'

Jim Goodnight: American billionaire and CEO of SAS – a statistical analysis institute.

Strategy Solutions

A. What can you as a family member do?

— Show leadership in every situation – and choose your battles. Genuine approachability will go a long way to finding out the gossip and getting support workers to go above and beyond for your person with disability. If you need to make a complaint, decide whether it's best to raise it in the moment or put it in writing once you're calmed down. Having things in writing is essential for ongoing issues.

— For all those whose workplace is their home (i.e. every mum or dad) – your staff being your partner and/or other kids, as well as the support workers who support your people with disability – your office is the study and the boardroom the dining room table; it really isn't that much different.

— Here are four things to consider when managing your family:
    1. What are your core values as parents, or as a family?
    2. Have you been able to organise the best available support workers to come into your home?

3. Have you delegated chores to family members, so all can share the load?

4. Do you get regular respite, so you can recharge your batteries and maintain your other relationships? Remember what flight attendants say when they give their pre-flight safety speech. If an oxygen mask is needed, and falls from the ceiling, please place the mask on yourself first, before helping others. You are no good to anyone if you're completely exhausted, unwell or overwhelmed.

— I used to hate it when extended family members or strangers used to assume that we 'regular' kids were somehow missing out on their parents' love and attention when they had to endure a sibling with a disability. I always felt my life was enhanced by having such siblings. We all learnt compassion, flexibility, and a true understanding of diversity by having people with disability in our family (and I had three such siblings!). In fact, I would say that I feel rather blessed.

There are times when your thoughtfulness, your small kindness, will literally change a person's life.

B. What can support workers and their providers do?

— Three ways to be a leader in your workplace, regardless of your title: be friendly, be generous and be brave

— Download my 'Disability Leadership Regardless of Title' PDF at <http://www.mzuritraining.com.au/resources.html>.

Additional Resources

— 'Interactive Care – Resources', Mzuri Training, <http://www.mzuritraining.com.au/resources.html> to read the following linked articles:

1. The Puzzle of Leadership – by Julienne Verhagen

2. Bradberry, T 2017, '10 Habits of Super Likeable Leaders', Huff Post, <https://www.huffingtonpost.com/entry/10-habits-of-super-likeable-leaders_us_591c78fde4b0a8551f3f84ee>.

3. Middlemiss, N 2015, 'How to handle being a young HR manager in an older office', HRD, <https://www.hcamag.com/hr-news/how-to-handle-being-a-young-hr-manager-in-an-older-office-196593.aspx?keyword=age>.

4. HCA 2014, 'HR should look for 'Shrek' when recruiting', HRD, <https://www.hcamag.com/hr-news/hr-should-look-for-shrek-when-recruiting-192981.aspx>.

Chapter 6

Boredom Kills – Everything

I don't like being bored. Really bored.

I like to be active and involved wherever possible. Sometimes I'm seriously, deeply bored, to the point where I want to explode – but I can't, so I escape by going to sleep.

This happens just about every day. What brings me out from the deep dark hole of boredom is vocalising (speaking with my own voice) a proper conversation with someone (about me!). I like travelling, music, being outside and feeling the sun on my face and the wind in my hair, and being with people who see through my disability.

Scott Clough

German philosopher Arthur Schopenhauer said, 'The two enemies of human happiness are pain and boredom.' Pain, we can all understand, is an enemy to happiness. It saps our energy, our patience, our coping mechanisms and it can affect our whole being. Even though many people with disability are often in regular pain, it's the latter of the two I want to explore: boredom.

I'm passionate about this theme: 'Boredom Kills – the Mind, the Body, and the Spirit (Interactive Care is not a luxury, it's a right).'

Boredom causes behavioural changes; it damages a person's sense of spirit and it can actually affect the physical body. It can stress your adrenal glands, disturb your sleep patterns and damage your self-esteem. The more prolonged, continuous and regular the boredom is, the greater the damage that can happen.

Boredom is not the same as just not doing much. When we're sitting in front of a television we're not doing much, but we're following something, engaging in what's happening on the TV and decompressing. We're usually in control of which room we want to sit in, which show we want to watch, the level of volume, and how we are sitting to watch it.

Meditation is a form of doing nothing, but the pursuit of a still mind or running visualisations keeps our attention focused and is not the same as being bored.

The boredom I'm talking about is when you spend at least 1–2 hours a day – or 2–3 times a day – where you have no choice where you are or what is going on around you, and there is quite simply nothing to do. No stimulation (or poor stimulation) that becomes like white noise. This is what many people – those with intellectual disabilities and those who are treated as though they have intellectual disabilities – have to endure day-in and day-out.

In some group homes, few support workers make the leap from being caring and hardworking, to ensuring that the clients are never sitting there doing nothing (unless it's a specific 'nothing' that they have chosen to do).

I'm not talking about a deliberate choice to do something relaxing. Scott loves to sit outside and just feel the breeze on his face, and being in the sunshine is heaven to him. One man in a home I'm familiar with loves to play video games. He's not physically doing much, but he's actively engaged with the games he is playing. Another man absolutely loves jazz music and will be happy listening to it for hours. What I'm talking about is all the rest of the time when someone is left doing nothing.

A few years ago, two professionals went to a meeting at an activity centre, where people with disability pay to attend, usually five days a week, to learn life skills, gain experiences, explore hobbies, play games and be challenged and stimulated each day. When they arrived, it was just after lunchtime and the clients were mostly all in one room. They were in wheelchairs, facing out, away from each other (if you can imagine pushing a wheelchair into a room and leaving it where you pushed it). They were all essentially facing separate walls.

Walking into the room, all the professions could see were backs of heads. One lady turned her motorised chair around and said hello. The rest couldn't see who had come into the room. No staff greeted them at the front entrance or knew they were there, even though they were on time for their meeting. They sat there with the clients in this room for about 20 minutes before anybody came in and noticed the guests were there, and ushered them into the office for the meeting.

Now, let's not even go into the security issues of this situation, or the lack of supervision for the clients who could have had a seizure, started choking on leftover food or such. Let's just ask: what were all of these clients doing for that 20 minutes? Absolutely nothing.

I don't want to criticise the staff too much here, because I know what they would have been doing. After spending an hour helping each client to have lunch, they then spent the next hour or so taking people who needed the toilet or personal care to a separate space where they could have dignity and the needed equipment to assist them. Two staff are usually required to attend to each person, and there are usually two change rooms in a centre, which leaves no one left with the rest of the clients while they're attending each person of focus.

The general routine is that they'll bring someone back into the room and think, 'Okay, who's next?' This is the drill. It's one of those disadvantages of having a group of people with disability all together who require manual handling to help them toilet and/or change clothes.

The duty of care is an important aspect here though. Multiple clients were left unsupervised like this, with their backs to each other, facing the walls. It was silent, but it didn't have to be. They could've had music, the radio or a video going for them. They could have been facing each other and even put into groups where those capable could have had conversations with each other. The window blind could have been up and the window open. None of these things require extra staff, time or money – just caring thought and an intention for the clients to be active or stimulated whenever possible.

The fact is that at each lunchtime in most activity centres where there are people with severe disabilities, you'll have up to 15 people in a room and 2–4 staff to help follow the routine. So for up to 2 hours every day, the people with disability all sit there doing nothing.

I know that in Scott's previous activity centre, they often had the radio on during lunch. Of course you can't have consensus with 15 people, so usually only those who had speech got to influence the type of music played. Staff would often touch base with these individuals during the changeover to the next person: 'Are you okay, John? Everything good with you, Scott?' But there's no time for meaningful conversations. The staff are working their butts off but the clients are bored, bored, bored.

As a result of years and years of this happening every day at his various day centres, Scott just switches off after lunch. He doesn't have a post-lunch nap, he has a 1½-hour sleep, because there's nothing else to do. It breaks my heart.

In fact, going to sleep has become Scott's way of dealing with things that are boring, annoying or frustrating. He just nods off and has a power nap. This can happen at quite inopportune or frustrating times! It also wreaks havoc on Scott's sleep cycle. The staff wonder why he wakes up in the middle of the night, wide awake, and I'm sure it's because he's been asleep half the day.

To give some comparison for you, let's have a look at the way most people would raise a new puppy. Fido would get walked daily, get patted and stroked and cuddled, and he'd play outside. At night Fido would get to chew on some toys, with lots of 'aww you're so cute' and 'good dog' all day. Fido would know he is loved and get to give sneaky little doggie kisses to show his affection.

But many people in supported accommodation go for days without spending any real time outside, or playing or exercising. And while some staff are wonderfully affectionate, clients rarely get actual cuddles or much opportunity to express their gratitude and affection for others.

People with disability, either due to lack of family or lack of funds, often have no private health insurance; they have very little say in what medical treatments or medications they're given. And, as already mentioned, many do not get any say in who makes up their medical and/or therapeutic team.

Some children and adults don't have one person in their lives that they belong to and when they do see friends or family members, because it's infrequent, most visits are reduced to niceties rather than quality conversations. How often do we have time for a real conversation about what someone might be feeling or what goals they want to achieve?

If you're their main carer or disability support worker, you're their main source of connection to another person. Sometimes you're their only family. They live with other disabled people and do activities with other disabled people. Self-advocates who can get into the workforce love it so much, but not just because of feeling empowered and earning wages; it's about being out there with regular people, having regular conversations and connections with others.

Scott goes through the boredom routine every day, even though he's in a well maintained home with good staff. He gets up when staff are ready to get him up. He needs to be changed and dressed for the day before being transferred (using a sling and ceiling-mounted hoist) from his bed to his wheelchair – all before staff can even give him a drink of water. Breakfast is usually the same each day because the staff know what he likes, and then off he goes to his activity centre for the day. Scott travels by maxi taxi (wheelchair accessible) and the same taxi drivers tend to do the shifts each day.

Scott is placed in the back of the taxi, so drivers don't tend to talk to him, and because he doesn't speak I've noticed that most of them don't even say hello to him! They just load him into the taxi, like a sack of potatoes. Scott is therefore quite isolated as he's transported to his day centre.

It doesn't have to be boring. He has an iPod connected to his wheelchair, so he can listen to audiobooks and music during his journeys – but though we've tried everything to have consistency, not having the same support workers work with him each morning means that he rarely gets to listen to an audiobook in order or within any realistic timeframe. Months can go by where they just forget to turn it on, or the staff at the other end don't turn it off and the battery goes flat.

Scott then gets to his day centre to participate in whatever activity is designated for that day – including the excruciatingly tedious lunchtime routine – before being transported back home again by another busy taxi driver who doesn't talk to him.

In 2006, there was a series of protests and news articles about three Australian zoos having nine Asian elephants imported from Thailand into their brand new state-of-the-art enclosures. Melbourne Zoo was creating a 'walk' so the elephants could transfer from one enclosure to another, which included long plant-filled and water-filled arenas. But instead of it getting good publicity, there were many protests. People were fighting for animal liberation.

Even though the protestors acknowledged that the elephants would be well cared for in these new enclosures, the argument was that elephants are incredible animals. They have traditions and communicate with each other, living in communities with specific gender roles; they grieve for their young, they use tools and work together to help each other. The main complaint was that these beautiful creatures would be bored in this gilded cage with nothing to do.

An International Fund for Animal Welfare campaigner tried to ensure agreement with the zoos that if the elephants started to show behaviours that displayed stress or boredom, then they needed to provide enrichment programs for these animals or move them to an open range zoo.[20]

One night, my mother and I were watching a news item about the elephants on the television. The complaint was how cruel it is to force them into long term boredom. Mum got quite emotional, exclaiming, 'Yes, but that's what's happening to Scott. What about my son? He's bored to death every day of his life.'

No matter how much we try, boredom is a big part of Scott's life. I've visited Scott at one of his day centres at 2.30 pm, when I've asked what Scott would usually do now. They've said, 'Well, his taxi will be here at 3.15, so there's no real time to do anything.' This is so frustrating, and it just goes on and on, and boredom reigns.

Sometimes the frustration is not from not doing anything, but from doing the same things over and over again. Special education, while terrific in many ways, are often places where, for example, sixteen year old people with disability are still going over their ABCs. The prevailing belief that people with disability take longer to learn things is not always true. Scott, for example, has an amazing memory.

The boredom can also come from us 'carers' and family members, keeping our charges 'occupied'. It drives me nuts to see the same childlike movies being shown over and over again in group homes. I know that some of the clients really like them (I'm a sucker for *The Sound of Music* myself!) but once or twice a year is enough. I know of places that play Sesame Street and the Wiggles every day, over and over again. *The Sound of Music*, *Mary Poppins*, *The Lion King*, *Toy Story* and *Frozen* – they're all fabulous movies, but if you have to watch them every week of your life for 40 years, it can be enough to send anyone into a rubber room. If one person likes this, then let's work with that, trying to expand their interests over time. But if these children's shows are being played in the main living area, then everyone has to put up with it.

Remember, people with limited mobility can't just get up and walk away. They have to grin and bear it.

I usually get the standard objections regarding this notion of boredom. The first is about having the time and the second is about not having the funds to create all these amazing opportunities. It takes consistency of staff, and innovative ideas and support from managers, and a budget and energy and … oh, it's just too hard! If you're a support worker in a group home, you have to take care of showering, toileting, cleaning, cooking and feeding. You don't get time to do all these activities, so clients have to sit there while the dinner gets cooked and the dishes are done.

Well, I get that. There are definitely busy times when those tasks have to take priority. But I put it to you that for the rest of the time, as a support worker, it's actually your job to plan the time and budget the money (if needed) to be interactive with your clients.

The opposite of boredom is to be engaged, stimulated, learning, laughing and living life to the max. The learning can be academic, daily skills or hobbies. Any form of learning, being challenged and socialising with others will pay off hugely in their sense of self and love of life. Is it possible for your clients to be involved with higher learning? Ask yourself – ask them. Let's stop the boredom, because it kills everything: the body, the mind, the spirit.

Strategy Solutions

A. What can you as a family member do?

— As parents, we don't always get our children involved in cooking meals – we know they'll learn eventually. But that time in the kitchen can become a special bonding and learning time for you and your person with disability. They can use all of their senses, spend time with you and know more about what's happening for dinner than their siblings!

— If their goal requires more substantial funds, have you considered crowdfunding? It's quick and effective. Even a Facebook post about what your person with disability wants to achieve can get amazing support.

B. What can support workers and their providers do?

— In terms of specific activities, even just one fun activity a week would be 52 times that they get to do something interesting each year.

— It's about how you use the time that you've got. If you're cooking dinner and you've got three people to supervise while you do it, include them in the task. If they can't physically assist, involve them. 'We're making this chicken cacciatore tonight, so what goes in chicken cacciatore? Chicken! Do we want to have it with rice or potato?' Involve them in aspects of preparing a meal, even if they can't physically do it. All the sensory smells are particularly interesting if your client is missing a sense like sight or sound. Let them smell the onions cooking and hear them frying.

— If you're watching the football on television, don't just stick them in front of it. Talk to them about the footy teams, who's winning and what's happening. Grab their footy team scarf to wear during the game, make popcorn and sing the team song during the ad breaks! Just get involved!

— As far as activities requiring money goes, let's teach them about saving – or at least plan it out for them. There's validity in saving across a few weeks for something special at the end of the month.

C. What can we do as a movement, with and for people with disability?

— Sporting clubs, scouting groups, drama clubs, recreation centres, GymbaROOs, and all other community businesses: open your doors to children with disability, adults with disability, and families that happen to include a person with disability. Make it as broad or specific as you like. Take it slow at first, so you don't get overwhelmed, then watch every participant benefit from the inclusion of people with diverse abilities.

— Educators in schools – it is your obligation and responsibility to do everything to can to include people with disability into your school. Be bold, take the initiative, and make it work!

Additional Resources

— Zev, S 2016, '19 Great Things To Do When You Are Disabled And Bored', Confined to Success, <https://confinedtosuccess.com/great-things-to-do-when-you-are-disabled-and-bored/>.

Chapter 7

Safety! – With Life

I can't talk about safety. My mind goes to the traumatic times when I was not safe, and I was really hurt, and it's too hard to talk about.

But I can talk about having a life! Trips to America, doing courses with good people, really flavoursome restaurant food at special dinners and family events, and knowing that my dog Jimmy is here with me.

Scott Clough

Safety, safety, safety! This is not a paranoid, overprotective, OHS slogan. It's a cry for help. A desperate plea for someone to please do something to protect our most vulnerable citizens from carelessness, apathy and deliberate cruelty. So, safety, safety, safety! It's a very real concern.

There are two parts to this chapter, forming a delicate balance if we want to enable people with disability to have meaningful lives. Nothing is more important than being safe, but we also want to have a life. This theme is called 'Safety First – But Quality of Life a Very Close Second (Let's be safe, but let's live too)'.

Fact: abuse and neglect for people with disability is rife throughout Australia and the world.

In January 2018, one hundred medical professionals signed an open letter to the Prime Minister of Australia calling for a royal commission into the abuse and neglect of people with disability in Australia. One hundred professionals spoke out and put their livelihoods, their careers and their names on the line to implore the government to at least look into what's going on and put something in place to address the damage they were encountering far too often in their daily practice.[21]

Because the NDIS is coming into play, the government has assured us the checks and balances put in place will be enough. But those in the know don't feel that goes far enough. It doesn't address the current exploitation of people with disability, or crimes of the past. There is no statute of limitations on murder, rape, sexual abuse, neglect to the point of death and permanent further disability. I believe that only a royal commission will have any hope of uncovering the destruction of spirit that has happened to so many people.

Child abuse and elderly abuse are both so repugnant, and people with disability can be included in either of those categories. They all share a burden of proof which is incredibly unfair. There is little to assist them in a conviction, and usually no corroborating evidence. People are prone to dismissing things that children say, and some elderly are too frightened to tell family what may have happened to them. For many of the disabled, not only do they have both of those issues to deal with, but if they are non-verbal, and cannot express what has happened to them, is can be virtually impossible to get any form of justice.

My contention is that regardless of criminal convictions or supportive evidence, the research suggests that people with intellectual disabilities, or those without speech, do not tend to make up stories about abuse. They at least need to be believed and supported when a complaint is made.

Because of their limitations, it's often not a spoken disclosure, but changes in behaviour that raise suspicions of abuse. People with disability who don't speak, or have limited speech, display tell-tale signs that are quite clear when you look for them. The problem is that we're not looking for them, or staff are so busy with day-to-day stuff, that they're not aware enough. Group homes are staffed with many casuals, and home-based carers are often casual, so they don't get to know someone well enough to have that perspective to be able to see differences in behaviours.

It gives me chills to think of how many people have never been supported at all through their abuse, because it's never been discovered.

And when it is suspected, often it doesn't change anything for the victim. One mother said to me not long ago that she's absolutely sure her son had been sexually abused, about a year earlier. When I asked her about it, she mentioned that her son's behaviour suddenly changed and he became pseudo-sexual towards her while showing real distress. She commented that he acted like this for several weeks before she noticed a slow return to normality for him.

When I asked if she'd said anything to anyone, she shrugged her shoulders. 'I've got no evidence. I have no idea when or how or who – so what can I do?'

For the uninitiated, most homes and supported accommodation utilise either reliable visiting support, or permanent workers who do their regular shifts. Having the same people each day brings consistency, long term progress, and relative security for the clients – assuming those regular staff are quality workers. When they are on leave, or ill, or have left and have not yet been replaced, most providers have a pool of regular casuals hired by the organisation, vetted by the provider and often having spent time in the relevant homes, so they are at least familiar with the clients.

When institutions and group homes get overwhelmed and cannot fill shifts, they call in the agency casuals. These are support workers who – bless their hearts – get called up at a moment's notice and go where they're told. Often, due to the late notice, things are in a shambles when they turn up and they're thrown into the deep end, looking after people they've never met before. I know because I've done it.

I know what it's like to rock up to a household and you have no real idea what you're walking into. It's nerve-wracking. You don't know any expectations, the client's emotional state, the family dynamic or if there are any behaviours of concern you'll have to cope with. Still, in a family home, someone is usually there to at least introduce the client, explain the basics and even show them what to do to orient them.

The situation in group homes is not always so accommodating. There are many times when casuals take over a shift with little or no transition, training or even handover.

Having casual staff in any house on a regular basis is very troubling. When I think of Scott being cared for, shift after shift, by people who don't know him, it's so concerning. They won't know how he expresses pain, when he's having an asthma attack or when he's having an epileptic seizure – any one of which could be catastrophic for him. Even the little things like how he needs to be positioned in bed for a comfortable night's sleep, how he must have lots of liquid with his meals or he could choke, or how he best takes his medication.

These are all things that a first or second-time visitor to his home can't possibly know.

Most supported accommodation providers have strict rules about meal plans, medication double-checking, and dignity with manual handling. After seeing the realities that can come from a lack of these policies in other countries, I'm so very pleased we have these procedures here, but they are not always followed.

Every housing facility has to employ casuals at some point, but people tend to develop relationships with families when they go regularly to homes, so they can request regular shifts and things can settle into a routine. Support workers feel obligated and committed to attending their client, and rarely miss shifts. The larger the group home or institution, the less personally invested staff can become. Also, the more problematic a home is (due to poor management, the environment or the clients), the more people take unexpected breaks and sick leave, and the more often providers have to use agency staff. While things will happen occasionally, I think it's a telling sign if a group home or institution seems to constantly employ a lot of casuals.

Of course, the greater the number of workers supporting a person with a disability, the greater the chance of mistakes, injuries and abuse. It makes sense that if you have 1–2 people looking after you, the likelihood of being mistreated by one of them is much lower than if you have 30 different staff members who are supporting you. While Scott's group home has about 10 regular support workers, when it comes to the number of casual staff he endures, 30 is not an exaggerated number. This is the reality for my brother and many people living in group homes.

The risk is increased not just from the numbers, but also from the increased anonymity, and decreased personal investment into and knowledge of the client. Irregular shift workers are also less likely to pick up on behavioural changes if someone is ill, injured, upset or intimidated.

The Disability Services Commissioner made a statement in the 'Our Year In Review' document for 2016–17. He reflected that one of the major issues with support workers putting in complaints about concerns of abuse of their clients is that they refuse to be named. They feared losing their jobs, in retribution by the organisations they work for. Support workers, by calling the DSC, enact the 'zero tolerance' of abuse that providers plaster all over their websites. But the reality is, these workers are calling the

DSC as a last resort, because they ether don't feel they can report to their management, or have reported it and it's not been acted upon, and they are terrified of being labelled a trouble-maker. As the DSC report attests, this was the case for every single support worker in 2016–17 who alerted the commissioner to a possible abuse or neglect situation.[22]

Disability service providers are not praising and working with staff who raise suspicion of abuse. It's obviously a very real problem. This is shameful behaviour by providers. When support workers fear for their jobs – real or imagined – when doing the right thing, something is very wrong.

Safety First

I want to talk about the many different forms of safety, or lack thereof. People with limited mobility usually have a cane, a frame or a wheelchair to assist them getting around. Scott lives in his manual wheelchair, and there are many aspects of life in a chair that can have safety concerns.

Pushing Scott through doorways in his chair – without bashing his arms, elbows, fingers or toes on the way through – is a constant problem. I've done it to him myself, so I understand how easily it can happen, but he's received many injuries this way. Safety first.

Forgetting to put the brakes on a wheelchair can cause horrendous injuries. Scott has literally rolled across a footpath, over the curb onto a main road at a busy bus stop, and tipped right over onto his front, face and arms. He received a deep cut above his eye, was black and blue from his shoulder to his wrist, and had a fluidic impact cyst covering his entire elbow which took months to heal. Safety first.

Then there are the little details that matter: conscientious placement during a transfer so that the person with disability is sitting in their wheelchair properly, carefully putting on shoes so toes are not bent or squashed, shoe laces done up, shaving carefully, ensuring enough warm clothes in winter, taking layers of clothing off when the day heats up, ensuring that people have been toileted often enough during the day, offering enough drinks to people between meals, etc. Safety first!

Accessible transport, particularly maxi taxis, and the lack of expertise or effort to secure people in wheelchairs safely is a real sticking point for me. Taxi drivers are forever securing the anchors to the wrong part of the wheelchair, or they criss-cross the straps (incorrectly thinking this is safer). They don't bother removing front trays, which can be deadly if having to brake suddenly. Some taxi drivers consider that because the person is secure in their wheelchair, and the wheelchair is strapped to the vehicle, that they don't need a seatbelt. All information on accident prevention says this is incorrect, and they require a proper seatbelt in the vehicle, just like anyone else.

Scott gets upset with me when he's being incorrectly loaded into a taxi or van. He rolls his eyes as if to say 'here we go' as I start telling them to undo the straps and attach them correctly, remove the tray and put a seatbelt on him! Many do not like being told that what they've been doing for the last five years has been wrong, but my brother's life is at stake every time he gets into a vehicle, so I don't care. I do try to be nice, but I don't compromise his safety. There are good ones out there, and they can really make our day – you just need to be vigilant!

Another general gripe about supported accommodation is the amount of times people complain of the support workers not knowing what their family member has been doing that day (or the previous day) when you call or visit that evening. They often have no idea because 'they've just come on duty', or they 'haven't checked communication dairy or schedule yet'. It happens all the time in many places.

As a result, not only can we not talk to our family members easily about what they've done that day, but the staff can't either. This rules out the most normal, relevant conversation with the clients for that entire day or evening. (Not to mention noting medical or other issues that are relevant to actively supporting their clients.)

This handover and communication is vital, particularly if the clients cannot tell you themselves what they've been up to that day, and is essential to good, interactive support. A minimum of three people are responsible for each handover – the staff member handing over, the one taking over and their manager, ensuring it's being done quickly but thoroughly, every shift change.

Sometimes the greatest risks to our safety come from the people we least expect. That misuse of authority and betrayal of trust that occurs when a practitioner becomes a perpetrator is horrendous. A senior doctor at a major hospital was strongly suspected of abusing his (primarily disabled) patients during appointments in his consulting room. The hospital board, instead of taking decisive action, put a roster in place to ensure he was not alone when seeing patients.

This effort to curtail his behaviour proved ineffective and he was eventually stood down after repeated accusations of inappropriate conduct. His clients, though, were never warned, questioned or encouraged to report any abuse by this practitioner. We'll probably never know how many people have been profoundly affected by his depraved behaviour.

I have recently re-certified my general first aid and CPR training, as well as asthma response and anaphylaxis training. I'm sure that most providers are vigilant in ensuring their staff are up-to-date as well, but two areas about safety regarding first aid concern me.

One is that as most people with disability live at home, there is no guarantee that their family members are up-to-date with their first aid. First-response and CPR practices have changed dramatically over the years.

Secondly, while most support workers are up-to-date, I don't see a lot of evidence of people being proactive with their training in real situations. Time and again, people underestimate the need for rest, ice, compression and elevation for injuries and swelling. People don't call ambulances quick enough and don't know the right thing to tell the ambulance to get the urgent help required. One girl I know has a very high pain tolerance, which is often confused for not being in pain at all, feeding her family's frustration at the continuous lack of pain relief she gets offered.

There are many aspects to 'safety first', but being ever vigilant for signs of abuse is, of course, crucial. The Royal Commission into Institutional Responses to Child Abuse released findings that told of very clear signs of abuse observed, and the lack of anything being done about it. Signs of abuse include:

— sudden changes in behaviour

— not wanting to go to a certain place or be with a particular person

— displaying unusual sexual behaviour

— becoming 'clingy' and wanting to stay with you

— not wanting to be alone

— unusual aggravation or anxiety.

These could all be indications that they're upset, confused or anxious about something that has happened to them. If you notice anything like this, you must note any telling behaviours and report them to your manager. If you don't get anywhere with management, call the Disability Services Commissioner.

As mandatory reporters, school teachers have actions they're required to do, actions they have the option to do, and actions (or inactions) that they cannot take. An important thing to note is that the burden of proof is never solely on the person making the complaint. It's not a teacher's job to be 100% certain of abuse or neglect before reporting it, or whether it's serious enough to go to the authorities. If they have a reasonable suspicion, they must report it up the line.

I raise the motion now that all permanent disability support workers, and their managers, should become mandatory reporters. This would introduce compulsory training, increase the likelihood of swifter reporting and perhaps improve organisational protections for reporters. Anyone want to second the motion?

The Disability Services Commissioner also stated in the Our Year In Review that:

> One consistent theme identified was that service providers appear focused on gathering conclusive evidence to substantiate an allegation or basing their decisions on whether Victoria Police charge someone with criminal offences. Services should instead focus their internal investigations on determining the likelihood that the incident occurred, and identifying strategies to prevent a similar incident from recurring. The experience of the person with a disability and other service users who had been involved should be paramount.[23]

People with disabilities who are able to disclose that they've been hurt, abused, or neglected need to hear these words: 'We believe you. We're sorry that this has happened, and we are taking steps so that this doesn't happen to you or anyone else again.' Whether the provider is the local council, accommodation provider, activity centre, educational facility, workplace, sporting club, dance class – wherever something has gone wrong, this is what we need to hear from whomever allowed it to occur on their watch.

Instead, I know of several cases of serious incidents where no acknowledgement of believing the victim, no apology, no acceptance of responsibility and no changes implemented to ensure improved standards of care have been given.

The second part of this chapter may seem like a contradiction, which is why I've deliberately put them together. As you can tell, I'm all about safety – but it is also important that a person's freedoms and opportunities are considered when making decisions that affect a client's life. That consideration is about their quality of life.

Quality must be a consideration too. In other words, safety comes first, but quality of life a very close second. Compared with limiting a person's enjoyment of life, some risks are worth taking. Here are several examples to demonstrate.

If someone has trouble eating a certain type of food, there is a risk that they might choke and that is a scary thing. But if you weigh up this risk versus having to be fed pureed food for the rest of their life – a balanced, considered choice is needed.

I teach occupational health and safety in my leadership workshops. The risk management table is a good guide and used to safeguard people from harm. But it's one thing to tie up loose power cords on the floor to avoid the risk of tripping or receiving an electrical shock; it's quite another to remove all electricity from the house because someone might get hurt!

It's all about taking manageable risks. Tradies climb ladders, walk on roofs and swing hammers every day. Surgeons manage risk during every operation. In other words, risk management is not only about stopping bad stuff from happening, it's also about safely making great stuff happen!

My favourite student as a teacher aide was the gregarious 'Merry' (short for Meredith). She had such a spark about her and a love of life that I will never forget. Every week we took our class swimming, but Merry was never allowed to go. All her file said was that it was a 'safety concern'. After being there for over a year, I asked her charge nurse about it and we discovered the reason was because she had a seizure as a one year old baby and was labelled an epileptic. As such, it was against medical advice for her to swim, in case she had a seizure in the water – even though there was no record of Merry ever having another seizure, and many epileptics swim regularly. (Scott is a severe epileptic but he swims twice a week!)

Another example of safety versus life includes Scott. One of his favourite snacks is potato crisps. While he does love his 'chippies', when having a meal plan assessment a speech therapist noted that a support worker had seen Scott coughing a couple of times when he was given too many chips at once. Possibly a choking hazard? Yes. So, the conclusion was that Scott was never allowed to have potato chips again. Ever! This all-or-nothing approach to risk, I believe, is missing balance.

Johnny is a young resident of a group home near Brisbane who also underwent a meal assessment after a staff member experienced him coughing during dinner and was concerned about him choking. The therapist noticed that, having a very high palate and narrow jaw, Johnny struggled to eat his meat if not chopped up small enough. The assessment stated to 'chop finely' all his meat and have it with gravy to keep it moist and help him to swallow.

We can only assume that one staff member read the assessment and surmised that they needed to vitamise his meat from now on. Vitamising food completely changes the texture and enjoyment of eating the meat. The natural progression for this was that, soon after, his entire evening meal was being vitamised. Meat, veggies, potato or pasta and gravy all pureed into a fine pulp! This worked well for the staff, as two other residents required their food to be vitamised also. And so this became the status quo for Johnny.

If a person with disability must have their food pureed, then let's vitamise each item separately, so there can still be some enjoyment of the meal. Can you imagine what putting everything together as one big mush for every meal does to a person's enjoyment of food? Even at formal social events, I've seen the support worker tip the entire plate of food into a vitamiser and slush it into a bowl for their client.

For Johnny, having his food reduced to mush was a very big deal, but he was not given a choice. And here's the kicker: no one told Johnny's family about it, so they had no idea until his dad visited at dinnertime, long after the assessment, and asked why his food was being vitamised. The support worker looked nonplussed and explained this was the way he always has it.

Managing risk (rather than always submitting to it) is not only important, but it can lead to adventure and fun! Marlena Ketene has cerebral palsy and she loves to sky-dive!

A slightly less extreme example was the day I brought Scotty to my bayside town last summer. It was a stinking hot day, topping 38 degrees, and I pushed his wheelchair to the sandy beach, where he could hear the waves and experience a cool breeze. It was heaven!

A storm was coming, and I kept reporting on the big dark clouds moving steadily across the bay towards us – but we just couldn't move because it was so great being where we were. Do we go yet? No – let's stay a bit longer. Now we've got to go or we're going to get drenched! Let's go!

Scotty was laughing and I was squealing as I pushed his wheelchair through the sand, up the alleyway and along the footpath to shelter. We were only seconds from being drenched.

The squalling rain became a wall of white wherever you looked. It was so loud you couldn't yell over it! And after such a swelteringly hot day, it was such an exhilarating and liberating and wonderful contrast. We both absolutely loved it. That's having a life!

When you go into a person's home – or at least their bedroom – has it been individualised? What says 'home' to you about your home? Personal touches in a house are so important, and having personal spaces that the client can invite others into at their discretion. Are the walls and rooms decorated in your client's group home? Are items such as hoists and wheelchairs out in the open and creating that hospital feel? And are items changed around, or has it looked the same for the past 20 years?

Welcoming spaces, such as a large couch in the lounge, an outdoor BBQ area and a decorating 'style' or 'theme', do wonders for making a house a home. Does the house smell nice or like cleaning product? Time to do an audit.

So, having a life has to be a very close second to safety – which, on balance, has to come first – but let's make sure everyone gets to enjoy variety, spontaneity, fun and adventure.

> *'A ship in the harbour is safe, but that is not what ships are built for.'*
>
> John A Shedd

Let's create opportunities to take the occasional risk, and get to have a life.

Strategy Solutions

A. What can you as a family member do?

— Put 'updating your first aid training' onto your to-do list!

— Part of our strategy with Scott was to let him explore. Remember Campbell Brown's comments? 'He'll toughen up!' Let your people with disability shine! Let them take risks – just manage them as best you can.

B. What can support workers and their providers do?

— Put 'updating your first aid training' onto your to-do list!

— Put 'managing risk' on your next staff meeting agenda. Are there times when we could raise the level of fun, learning and adventure by managing risk appropriately? Let's put a plan in place.

C. What can we do as a movement, with and for people with disability?

— Those people with disability – paralympians, sky-divers, world travellers and all of you doing amazing adventures where you manage risk – get the word out! Post your adventures on YouTube; tell your friends and let's set the examples for others.

Additional Resources

— 'Interactive Care – Resources', Mzuri Training, <http://www.mzuritraining.com.au/resources.html> to read the following linked article:

1. FACT SHEET: 5 Royal Commissions findings on abuse in group homes

Chapter 8

No Institutionalised Insanity

> *I don't like it when my home is run more like a hospital rather than a home. Some things that really cheese me off are all the staff coming and going (whether I know them or not) and blanket policies that stop things from happening for years and years – like how staff aren't allowed to feed me by hand, or put their hand over my mouth to help me vocalise. But that's the only way I can use my voice. There are other ways, like putting gloves on to help me use my 'voice'.*
>
> Scott Clough

No longer is it common practise to have hundreds of 'mentally retarded', 'spastic' and 'mute' people, and other 'idiots' living in large 'asylums': hospitals designed to treat these hidden-away 'sub-humans' with appalling 'diseases'. They had no right to choose any aspect of their lives; not the medications they had to take, not the medical procedures done for them and to them, and they certainly didn't have the right to vote or press charges on anyone doing them harm.

Today the living arrangements for most people with an intellectual disability, a visual or auditory impairment, autism spectrum disorder or other complex needs (e.g. those with cerebral palsy, spina bifida, thalidomide poisoning, Down syndrome, osteogenesis, motor neuron disease, muscular dystrophy, severe scoliosis, severe epilepsy, spinal injuries and brain traumas, etc.) are now certainly transformed for the better in many countries.

But regardless of intellectual ability of any person, we are still seeing institutionalised policies, ignorant practitioners, dominating managers and abusive situations occurring without consequences throughout Australia and the world.

In March 2017, Alison Branley wrote for the Australian Broadcasting Commission (ABC):

> A hundred years ago people with an intellectual disability were locked up in 'lunatic asylums'. Today they're still locked away, but it's just behind the walls of suburbia.[24]

In this chapter, I want to explore some of the ways many group homes, activity centres, aged care centres and other institutions have lost their way, forgotten their intended purpose and need a complete reboot. I call this theme: 'No More Institutionalised Insanity (Homes must be homes, not hospitals)', and I ask every staff member in an institutional setting or group home to please take note.

Interactive Care training could make the biggest difference to the lives of the people in all supported accommodation. With staff and management embracing the eight themes of Interactive Care, all the benefits of being grouped together could work for the residents rather than against them. It would ensure a whole different ball game.

People with disability need to be supported in a host of different ways. Some simply need their housework done for them, or help getting to places; some require daily social companionship and assistance with physical needs; others require round-the-clock care. Each case requires a co-ordinated effort.

Routine can be particularly important for many people. People with ASD, for example, feel much more comfortable when things follow a routine. People with visual impairments like to know what's happening around them; those who attend the toilet by time of the day need routine to keep comfortable.

Let's face it – most of us are creatures of habit, so routine can be reassuring, settling and can ensure that people receive the care they need. Having a spa bath every Sunday morning, going to a café day every Saturday afternoon, and Monday afternoons are for supermarket shopping. Friday night is 'take-out' night, Tuesday night is *Masterchef* night. Friday night football is a tradition in our home! We always put up the Christmas tree together at the start of December, and enjoy having a Christmas party to invite family and friends over.

These sort of routines and mini-traditions create family-style unity, a sense of belonging, and gives clients something to look forward to. They can also be changed if a special circumstance or event comes along.

While recognising the value of routine, it is vital that we don't allow routines to dominate the lives of the people being supported. When that happens they become more hospital-like, and more important than the people being supported – routines purely for staffing convenience rather than individual safety or group unity. These are the dictated times to get up, meal times and menus, cleaning routines, roster inflexibility, budget limitations, bathing time processes, and bedtime mandates. The clients should always come first!

While routine is important to some, spontaneity is the spice of life! It alleviates boredom, encourages individual choice, personalises and individualises events, and makes us feel alive.

— 'Let's not have the prescribed meal for dinner tonight. Who wants Chinese food?'

— 'Let's not all go to bed at 7 pm tonight – who wants to have a 30-minute impromptu dance party?'

This theme of 'No more institutionalised insanity!' relates to any group living arrangement that is overseen by professionals. Hospitals are a bit different here, because people are unwell there and must be strictly monitored and cared for because of their immediate medical needs. But aged care facilities, group homes, institutions, orphanages: take note.

Unless on the odd occasion that the client really wants this:

— No more having dinner at 4.30 pm and bed at 6.30 pm.

— No more showers at 3.30 pm and being put into PJs for the rest of the day.

— No more frozen pies and sausage rolls because it's Sat night, every Saturday night!

— No more having to come home from a theatre show, party or special event before it ends (or from a restaurant before dessert is even served) because the disability support worker has to be back for the end of their shift at 9 pm!

— No more communal clothing and communal bedding.

— No more fluorescent lights in homes (as they can really set off those with autism and/or light sensitivities.)

— No more anti-animal policies. The research is clear how much joy and comfort the right animal (dog, cat, rabbit, guinea pig, bird, etc.) can bring to people of all ages and abilities.

— No more industrial-strength chemical cleaners (unless required on the odd occasion in one specific location). The chemicals are damaging, the smell is nauseating, and it can affect the people living there in a host of negative ways.

But, I can hear some of you saying, support workers have to run the house, and routines are essential. This is true, and routines not only help things run smoothly, but many people with ASD, vision impairment or other conditions rely on routine to orient their world and keep anxiety at bay. It all depends on the clients and the situation. A balance between being task-focused and people-focused is necessary for ticking all the boxes.

One client in a group home I've visited often likes young children's shows. It helps keep her calm and lessens the amount of time she focuses on getting the staff's attention that she's so desperate to communicate to. It's been reported to me that for over a decade, no support workers were allowed to change the channel from the ABC children's shows. Part-time and casual support workers were literally threatened by the permanent staff with 'never getting any more shifts here' if they dared to change the channel.

Why? It's a behavioural strategy, keeping her busy so that they could do their household jobs and take care of the other residents. I can certainly see how this would be very useful on occasion and tempting to employ a lot of the time. The problem is that this negates the disability support worker's responsibility to engage with her. And the other clients living in the house had to put up with mind-numbing children's television in the main living area every day and night. It's their house too! (Not to mention it driving the staff around the bend at times as well!) I'm told they discovered support workers who chose not to work at that home again because of incidents like this.

Training is one area that relates to this. Support workers require a lot more than manual handling training. Here is a list of extra trainings that, over a period of time, I believe all permanent support workers should have access to:

— Cooking classes (so they can cook decent food for their clients and be aware of allergy and nutritional updates)

— Professional cleaning training (staff use strong chemicals, but they are not professional cleaners)

— Specialist disability first aid training (specialising in adapting to their specific client needs)

— Communication augmentation and assistive technology training (it breaks my heart to see people in all different situations with less communication than they could potentially have if organisations took the initiative to investigate alternatives)

— Podiatrist basic training (so someone in the house can safely cut finger and toe nails without having to wait six weeks to pay for a practitioner to come to the house to deal with a broken nail!)

— Communication apps and smartphone training (all teams should be in regular contact using easy apps, like WhatsApp or a closed Facebook group, to make messaging quick and easy)

— Six-monthly 'sit rep' meetings (a situation representation meeting where every client is discussed in detail. How do staff feel they're travelling? What is the state of their equipment? What initiatives can we start? What issues have the family raised that we need to discuss?)

Some facilities are doing some of these initiatives with great success, but I don't know any that are doing all of them – and many don't do any of the above.

The second area of note within this theme of 'no more institutionalised insanity' revolves around the way organisational and support worker priorities can affect the clients they're caring for. I want to give you several examples of where misplaced priorities have directly affected my brother Scott (involving several different providers over many years) and go on a rant about a pet hate I have in this category.

In transitioning Scott from living at home in the country to gaining access to his purpose-built small group home in the city, he was put on a waiting list. He was to live for at least 12 months in an old hospital-style institution in order to be on the list and wait until his new house was ready. It was a traumatic experience for him, and for us, that he had to move to such a facility. He had to cope with moving to a big centre with new staff and routines, attend a new day centre in a new city, and – being over 2 hours away – rather than seeing us daily, he only saw some of his family for two hours a fortnight.

His small bedroom was directly off the lounge and dining room – a large common area with dark brown industrial carpet – for one of the three wings of the facility. Clients whizzed in and out of the automatic sliding doors as you walked down the ramp, past the industrial kitchen to come into the lounge. Even though Scott was 22, what a big, scary and lonely change it must have been for him.

It could have been an exciting adventure. He seemed to love his new day centre, with terrific staff in an urban setting where he was taken around the shops to meet new people and have drinks in cafés! But the living arrangement was a different story.

Every time we went there we met different staff, and it always felt cold and unfriendly. I certainly didn't feel comfortable being there.

My mother knew this was part of the process and something Scott would have to endure, so she made only one standing request prior to agreeing to his move. As everything else in Scott's life would be changing, being visually impaired it would not be easy for him to orient himself, so his bedroom needed to be set out the exact same way it was at home. That way, he would at least know where things were and feel relatively comfortable in his own room. The configuration of his new room allowed for this and we set it up for him.

On our second visit, we walked into Scott's room and we noticed his entire bedroom had been reconfigured. Mum went to find someone and was told that they had moved it all a week ago to make it easier to use the hoist when lifting him in and out of bed. Mum was incredibly unhappy about this and asked them to move it all back again. Of course we were told it was a safety matter for the operator of the equipment, so that was the way it was staying.

I remember Mum getting quite upset and explaining to the staff that the setup of Scott's bedroom was the one thing that she got agreement on to keep the same as home. And without any consultation they had just moved it all.

'Have you even told Scott?' she cried. 'Have you at least told him why you've moved it around and helped him to know where everything is now?'

Of course they hadn't. That made them think a bit deeper about it and they apologised about not including Scott in the situation at all. There was no evil intent, just no consideration of the person involved.

There have been at least two occasions in recent years where Scott has sustained injuries severe enough to warrant late night trips to the emergency department of our local hospital. The second example is a very real problem with the current policy of most disability providers (and, I'm told, aged care facilities). The general rule is that once they are under the care of the nursing staff in a medical facility, the support workers are under no obligation to stay with them. They literally leave the clients there and go back to their workplace to resume their duties. I've heard of people with dementia left to their own devices and not having any food for days, people lying in soiled bedsheets for hours and being terrified at all the strange sounds.

I can concede that for some people with disability, while this would be a little scary or unsettling, they will be physically fine. Half of the clients who live in Scott's home, while I'm sure they'd appreciate having someone they know with them, can ask for what they need and would be okay. For others who have physical needs and/or a lack of communication (or severe dementia, or emotionally volatility when anxious), leaving them in the hands of incredibly busy nursing staff is a frightening prospect.

Scott literally cannot lie in a normal hospital bed without the possibility of falling out, or getting caught up in the side bars. He cannot eat or drink or sit up by himself; he cannot reach or push the panic button if he is in pain, or having a seizure, or he's thirsty, or scared. I would consider him to be seriously at risk if left unsupervised, even for a few minutes, in a busy hospital ward, and especially overnight. Yet that is exactly what the policy tells providers to do.

On the two occasions that this has happened, I was able to get to the hospital to be with him, so the disability support worker accompanying Scott was told by their manager to get back to the house. What would have happened if I wasn't there? Would the staff have left him there, alone? The official answer is yes – it's official state policy. In my book that is simply not acceptable.

The third example of policy over common sense care relates to Scott's diet. I visited one of his activity centres that he attended at that time, several days over a week. While I was there, I noticed that he had Vegemite, cheese and jam sandwiches, two chocolate puddings, potato chips and a 'popper' (cordial in a convenient little pop-top bottle) for lunch.

This didn't really raise any alarms at first, until I saw that he had the exact same lunch on all three days that I attended. On the third day I asked, 'Is this what Scott has for lunch every day?'

I got a big smile from the young girl supporting him. 'Oh yeah, he loves Vegemite and cheese.'

He's loved Vegemite and cheese since he was tiny, but bells went off in my head. Not only was it a boring lunch, but it was very basic food. White bread, margarine, processed cheese and cheap jam. No salad, meat, or real butter – nothing very nutritious at all. Remember, Scott has cerebral palsy and also osteoporosis. He's very thin and needs lots of protein-rich energy foods to build up his body and bones. The puddings were just full of sugar and the drinks were sugary sweet – and the whole lunch had no variety at all.

'Is this what he's been given for lunch and to drink every weekday for 11 years?' I asked.

'Well, that's all they give us,' was her reply.

At the time, I had long been annoyed at the group home's weekly meal schedule, which included party pies and sausage rolls every Saturday night for dinner. So we started asking questions about his diet. We discovered, for example, that all the residents in the house lived on low-fat milk and low-fat cheese because one of the residents had a weight problem. But Scott doesn't! He needs full-fat dairy and lots of high-quality, protein-rich foods.

At one point my mother mentioned the lack of drink he was given each day and asked, 'Even in summer, is one popper all that he gets to drink?'

The response was, 'No, we give him two drinks in summer.'

A speech therapist was eventually brought in to review Scott's diet, who decided that he required a variety of salads and cold meat sandwich fillings. He needed wholemeal bread with real butter, calcium-rich milk, cheese and real yoghurts each day.

I understand staff wanting to give Scott what he likes each day – and having a set routine makes things easy – but where was the priority of quality food, variety and choice? Scott paid decent money each fortnight for food and he deserved to have quality food for that.

I was in my local café a few months ago and a man in his thirties came in sat at the table next to mine. He had a disability and was accompanied by a support worker. He was directed to sit with a motion of the lady's hand who was accompanying him. She went to the counter to put in their order, then sat opposite him and read the paper while he sat there in silence, looking around the café. Of course I smiled and we have a quick connection. I tried to engage with the support worker but she made it clear she wasn't interested.

Eventually their food and drink came. She had eggs and bacon on toast and a large coffee; he had simple raison toast and a glass of milk. He and I had some pleasant conversations which she mostly ignored, in between looking at me suspiciously. They pretty much ate in silence and then she gathered him up and went.

What a fun outing for that lovely man! (Sorry, my sarcasm escaped for a brief moment!) Even though on paper this will look great ('Went to a café, and had yummy raison toast') it was full of missed opportunities, lost conversation, equal food, real choice or any chance for friendship. These subtleties are what concern me when I'm not there to ensure that Scott isn't just aimlessly walked around the shopping centre whenever he goes out. This is not Interactive Care.

My final point on the subject of staffing, apathy and institutionalised insanity is a personal beef I have. I realise not everyone will feel as I do, but it really irks me and if I can't get it off my chest in my own book, then when can I? This is an unapologetic rant about taking clients, as a group, at least once every week to the movies.

Please don't get me wrong. I love going to the movies. I'm an actress and a singer myself, and going to see plays, musicals and movies (including at the drive-in) can be a real treat. Plus, I've taken Scott to the movies myself, on special occasions or when he gets given tickets as gifts. He chooses what we see and what food he wants to eat while we're there, and it's great.

The positive socialising aspects include learning how to be quiet in that environment, the escape of extreme weather, and the physical feeling of the big sound and the big picture in the theatre (particularly for Scott, who's visually impaired).

But ... disability support workers are forever taking their groups of clients to the movies, sometimes several times a week, and I believe it should be discouraged as a regular activity.

Taking clients to the movies is a rort because there's no talking allowed in a movie theatre, no real socialisation, and you can't interpret the action for any client who is blind or deaf or needing the story explained in plain English to them. The snacks are expensive and unhealthy – and if the clients can't eat them, or can't afford them, they miss out on all the fun food.

If there is no 'companion card' accepted at the movie theatre, then clients have to pay for the support worker's ticket as well as their own, including the cost of transport. Support workers naturally take clients to a movie that suits the lowest common denominator (mentally or behaviourally) in the group. This means that more complex, intellectual, story-based or emotionally stimulating movies are seldom chosen.

When clients are taken to the movies, they are not outside in the sunshine, walking their dogs or playing board games with friends. They're not having a coffee in a local café where they get to chat with the owner and be part of the community. It's usually quite an anonymous exercise to sit in the dark and be quietly mesmerised for a couple of hours.

And here's why it's such a popular activity to do. Support workers get to do nothing for a couple of hours and get paid to watch a free movie! I understand it, and think it's fine on occasion, but as a general rule I'm calling it as a poor activity.

Let's look at if you decided to watch a movie (DVD, Netflix, Foxtel, etc.) at home instead. At home, support workers can interact with their clients while watching the movie. They can interpret what's happening, react vocally with/for them when exciting things happen, stop the movie at any time to attend to their needs. It saves the time, money and hassle of transport. The client/s can eat healthy, appropriate food, and be fed (or at least properly supervised with their eating) during the movie.

Support workers also get to watch the movie, but with interaction and involvement while attending to each individual's needs. You can also schedule films to cater for different tastes and intellectual levels in the group.

In my view, the only times clients should be taken to the movies are during extreme heat or cold, or for a special movie requested by the client. Otherwise, make a better choice.

So, I hear you ask, what do you do if you are an enthusiastic support worker who wants to initiate great activities, but it's either discouraged by the others you work with, or by the provider or family who employ you? Well, you have three things to consider.

1. With the NDIS coming to every Australian with the need for support, the person with disability is your actual employer, not anyone else – and that is where your loyalty needs to lie.
    9. Use this book! Use the Interactive Care model to encourage healthy and respectful discussion around this.
    10. If you can't make any headway where you are, leave. Find somewhere else before your enthusiasm starts to wane, and we lose you to a different industry.

Strategy Solutions

A. What can you as a family member do?

— With regards to hospital practises, it's official state policy, so if your person lives in supported accommodation there isn't much you can do in the short term. What you can do is *be there* if possible – and have an information sheet ready to go if you can't be there. Also, having a good relationship with the staff will create a better chance of being told if something happens.

B. What can support workers and their providers do?

— Get clients to come with you to answer the front door – after all, it is their house! Get them to welcome people (a good social skill), particularly if they're expecting a friend or family member to arrive.

— Welcome all guests and offer them a drink, giving introductions to others in the house. The clients could help prepare a drink for their guest.

— Rather than always putting clothes in the dryer, get the clients to help you hang washing out on the line. (This saves energy, lengthens the life of the clothes, teaches life skills, and it's an interactive activity which keeps the clients occupied)

Additional Resources

— 'Interactive Care – Resources', Mzuri Training, <http://www.mzuritraining.com.au/resources.html> to read the following linked article:

  1. FACT SHEET: 10 Essential Tips for Travelling with a wheelchair.

— 'Shut Out: The Experience of People with Disabilities and their Families in Australia' 2009, National Disability Strategy Consultation Report prepared by the National People with Disabilities and Carer Council, <https://www.dss.gov.au/sites/default/files/documents/05_2012/nds_report.pdf>.

— Branley, A 2017, 'Group home 'hell': Open letter calls for royal commission into treatment of people with disabilities', ABC News, <http://www.abc.net.au/news/2017-05-17/psychotropic-medications-in-group-homes-open-letter/8513664>.

— On Friday 11 January 2013, the Governor-General appointed a six-member royal commission to inquire into how institutions with a responsibility for children have managed and responded to allegations and instances of child sexual abuse. (Royal Commission into Institutional Responses to Child Sexual Abuse.)

— Morton, R 2014, 'Farewell to state care for the severely disabled', *The Australian*.

Chapter 9

Touchpoints of Care

> *I love this chapter. It's important to me and it makes me happy when staff ensure that I'm comfortable. There are lots of little things that need to be done properly or checked, and I really appreciate the care when someone checks everything.*
>
> *When I'm being put in my wheelchair, for example, I need my back and bottom to be put in the right place, my seatbelt to be done up tight, and my shirt to be pulled down at the back. I should have my ankle in a brace and my gel pads in my shoes; my feet need to be in the right position and my headrest needs to be screwed on tightly.*
>
> *That's a lot to think of, but I'm in my chair all day, every day, and it can be painful if it's not right.*
>
> *Scott Clough*

As a design and delivery specialist in leadership training, including customer service, I know that this theme is vital if we want to change the current status quo of disability support: 'Touchpoints of Care (Find moments to show you care, opportunities to serve, and to make magic happen).'

It's all about recognising the importance of customer service (and people with disability are your customers!) and creating opportunities to help and inspire them to learn, love, party, play, protest – and *try*. In today's fast-paced world of business, value for money and customer service are hugely important aspects.

I am constantly amazed at how, in the field of disability, this aspect of good business and best practice is generally still so lacking.

Let's look at this in more detail.

Jan Carlzon took over Scandinavian Airlines in 1981. This is an airline which had suffered a 30-million dollar loss, but within two years under Carlzon's new leadership, the airline became one of the best, and won 'Airline of the Year' from Air Transport World. What he said was they all knew how to fly planes, but if they wanted to be a successful airline, they had to learn how to fly people.

He focused on a business's only true assets: satisfied customers. Every single moment engaging with a customer was important. Of course, safety is paramount for an airline, and they had just bought a whole fleet of brand new aircraft. But did the public really care this? Not really. They cared about what Carlzon called the 'moments of truth'.

As customers, we care about how easy it is to find a flight and purchase a ticket. If we call the airline, how helpful are they? When we get to the airport, what is our check-in experience like? How quick and friendly are they at security? How smooth is the process? Are our on-board expectations met? These are the moments of truth. Carlzon took that problem-ridden airline and turned it around.

I believe just as relevant a concept in the caring professions. I call these moments our 'touchpoints of care'. There are so many opportunities for touchpoints of care, every time you interact with anyone.

It starts from the moment that the client being supported is awake until they're asleep. It's the way we say good morning, help them dress and set them up for the day. It's the way we place them in their wheelchairs, checking they're okay before giving them their choice of breakfast and drink. It's the little things previously mentioned, like having the clients answer their own front door, planning fun house events for the gang, offering a cup of tea to family members when they visit, and inviting them to occasional meals.

It's about delighting your clients, and great carers naturally think like this. They see opportunities for fun or involvement and then make it happen. These carers know that helping others to achieve their goals increases their own job satisfaction and creates a real sense of progress in their roles. They know that the endeavour of a pursuit – irrespective of how close to achievement one gets – is to know you are alive.

The second way we can implement touchpoints of care is to sweat the small stuff. I know there is a famous book out there about not sweating the small stuff – that the main things in life are what's important – and on a holistic lifestyle level, of course I agree. But when it comes to business, and any field work that involves children, the elderly, the injured or the disabled, I believe it's vital to be detail-focused. It's about sweating the small stuff for every person. Here are some examples.

One lady I know who is an involved aunty tells me her frustration that whenever she visits her niece, she can't help but see all of the little things that aren't right with how she is. Is she sitting in her wheelchair correctly? Is her headrest on the right angle? Is her face communication lever in the right spot and her COMPIC communication book on her tray where she can see it properly? Is her seatbelt done up in the right way, at the right spot? Is her t-shirt pulled down nicely at the back, or bunched up behind her?

Is her mobile phone in the holder where she can point to it when she needs to – and is it charged? Are her clothes her own, clean and co-ordinated? Are her teeth cleaned and her hair nicely done?

These are all touchpoints of care, and her aunty made the point to me that there has never been a time when everything was right.

In January this year, it was a stifling 39-degree day, and the air conditioning in Scott's home had broken down. The air conditioning company had bought in some industrial fans that had been on all day, and they did make a difference but it was still very humid in the house. Scott had been placed right in front of one of the big fans, as the moulded back of his wheelchair hugs his body and gives no relief in the heat. The staff were all doing the right things, trying to cope with the heat as best as possible.

Then I looked down at Scott with his t-shirt and shorts, and noticed he was wearing sheepskin woollen Ugg boots. I took his boots off and he had socks on underneath! I asked the disability support worker, 'Why does he have socks and Ugg boots on?'

'Oh,' the disability support worker said, 'just to be more comfortable for him.'

I took them both off his feet and the look of relief on Scott's face was priceless. I totally appreciate that Scott's support worker was thinking about his comfort, but what on earth was he doing with anything on his feet, let alone socks and Ugg boots? Ughh!

The third thing is to treat your people with disability as your customers, because they are! They're not the metaphorical pot plants that are decorating the room while you clean their house or make their dinner. They need and deserve to be communicated with and cared for as you go about your day. Any sort of opportunity you can find to make their life more interesting will be a benefit to them, their peers, yourself and the organisation.

A big but rewarding thing to do is to organise a holiday for them. It is possible to do, and if you find it all too difficult there are some terrific companies out there that do it all for you. I've organised overseas trips, local getaways, interstate holidays and day trips for Scott, whose physical requirements are super challenging. I've got a huge list of travel hacks for people who need to organise accessible travel, as I've learned the hard way what's essential to make magic happen. It's all about planning, so you can then be spontaneous! In fact, I find that making magic happen is the best part of the job.

Part of the touchpoints of care involves seeing the ability and the possibilities in our people with disability: what they can do, what they do feel, what they want to achieve, what they love or really enjoy.

Here's an example of how a different approach to exactly the same situation created a completely different experience for family. The first time we went to America, my mother, myself, our wonderful support worker (Rob) and Scotty travelled for just over three weeks. We flew home and got back to Scott's house, after three flights and an exhausting 30 hours of travel. We finally arrived at Scott's house, before Mum and I had to continue on our way with the taxi to get to my home. Now, it was organised that a staff member would be rostered on to be there for Scott when he arrived home, as the other residents would be out at their respective activity centres.

We arrived in the taxi after our extraordinary trip, and a casual staff member opened the door. A new support worker who'd never met Scott, who spoke little English, and who'd been haphazardly sourced by the house manager of the day. She didn't have any idea that he'd been away to America. We had to explain that we'd just come home from overseas and that Scott was desperate for a drink, then time on the toilet, then a shower, food and a rest in bed.

'Okay,' she said, 'I'll do that.'

The taxi was waiting and we had to leave him there, alone with someone who he didn't know, after we'd just spent nearly a month with him, full time. It was such an anti-climax for him, and though she may have been an experienced carer, it didn't seem like it to us, and we had no faith that Scott would have a pleasant or even safe experience in the house without us. It certainly wasn't the ideal way to end such a wonderful adventure.

The second time we went to America, I took Scott with our support worker for two extraordinary weeks away. Just as before, I got him back to his house via an accessible taxi, and one of his favourite, regular support workers was waiting for him. When we got to his house we saw a big colourful sign on the front door, saying, 'Welcome Home Scott!' We rang the doorbell and before the door had even opened we heard this huge 'Scotty!' from the wonderful Olivia, who ran to the door with hugs and a, 'Welcome home!' and, 'We've missed you!' She went on with, 'I've got a lovely shower waiting for you with all your yummy, nice bath gel, and I've got your favourite dinner on the stove ready to give you before anybody else turns up.'

Oh my gosh! What a difference – for him and for me – to be able to leave him knowing he was in such excellent hands. Being welcomed home like this was just one little thing, but it made a huge and memorable difference.

By sweating the small stuff and looking for opportunities for people to take ownership over the space that they live in, you can make it much more empowering and inclusive. I honestly don't feel that you have shut down community houses; you just need to run them better. You don't need to change the building; you just need to change the way they're being staffed and encourage the clients to have the power to be involved in their own homes, their own lives.

There are high-tech and low-tech ways of communicating with those who have limited speech – and an attempt at any system is better than none. You don't have to be a speech pathologist to talk to someone or attempt new ideas to communicate. I think support workers are often too intimidated to even experiment with ideas to improve communication with their clients. Try low-tech things first: pictures, symbols, auditory scanning and simple colour choices.

When it comes to high-tech, things are moving fast due to the gaming world. Be on the lookout for new things, because exciting advances are being made. 'Think to text' is coming. AlterEgo (intelligence augmentation) devices are being produced where your deliberate thoughts are recognised by wearing a headset and spoken/typed out! This is virtual mindreading – commercially available and affordable. I can't wait till it becomes available.

You see, regardless of labels, assessments and practitioners' opinions, we really have no idea what anyone's intellectual abilities are if they can't communicate – and it's not your job to define someone by those assumed limitations. Even with clear mental limitations, that's no reason to diminish offering choice.

In 2012, ABC America's *20/20* program did a special on a girl named Carly Fleischmann. She was from Toronto, Canada, and was diagnosed with autism and oral-motor apraxia at the age of two. She was thought to be so intellectually impaired due to her autism (ASD), and her lack of ability to communicate, that experts had written her off and recommended institutionalisation. She had never spoken a word, and had shown behaviours of concern like banging her head on the floor, screaming, hitting and even faecal smearing.

At the age of 10, Carly went over to a therapist's laptop in the family lounge room and typed HURT. Then she typed HEL…P. It was a breakthrough moment. Not only could she type letters and spell words, but she had reached out, and asked for help.

At first Carly resisted typing, and refused to perform for a camera or other therapists. But the family began some tough love for Carly. Whenever she wanted anything, she had to type it out. She got so much praise and reward after typing out her desires that her resistance softened. After several months she began typing in front of other people.

The ABC documentary, produced in August 2012, is still a fascinating one to watch, with the footage of Carly compelling. Now she is in her early 20s and her writing reveals her witty, honest and hilarious personality.[25]

She now conducts interviews with her pre-typed questions – her first one being with her celebrity crush, Channing Tatum.[26] Carly has also published her own website where you can experience what it's like for her, as a person with ASD, when she goes into a café. All the sounds and movements and colours and distractions are all at one loud level – she can't delineate and direct her focus on just some sounds like we can – which is why many people with ASD tend to cover their ears, flick their fingers in the light and rock and hum. It's all done to drown out the extraneous noise (and sometimes the pain they are experiencing) and be able to focus more on one thing.[27]

Your touchpoints of care with the people you work with can help stumble upon genuine breakthroughs. You never know.

I know I might seem a bit full-on about this – about making great stuff happen and creating and heightening occasions with people with disability. It really is for a good reason.

Find moments to show you care, opportunities to serve, and ways to make magic happen.

Strategy Solutions

A. What can you as a family member or support worker do?

— Ask yourself: 'How can I make magic happen today?'

— For example, can you give your child/client the experience of smelling fresh flowers? Some beautiful flowers once a month would add interest, aroma and a talking point. They'll keep for about ten days, plus you'll get to be in a place with beautiful, fresh flowers. It's win-win for everyone and it exceeds expectations.

B. What can you as a self-advocate do?

— If you're a person with a disability reading this book, and you're what we call a 'self-advocate', then you are the boss. You are the client and everybody else is working for you. So, you have the right to expect and demand decent customer service. If you don't get it, one of the great things about the NDIS here in Australia is that technically you can now say, 'I don't want you anymore. I want somebody else.'

Additional Resources

— O'Brien, J, 'Make a Difference: Support Valued Experiences – The Colouring Book', <http://www.centreforwelfarereform.org/uploads/attachment/597/make-a-difference-support-valued-experiences.pdf>

Chapter 10

Crucial, Meaningful Relationships

> *I love to be close to my family and friends and keep connected. I'm so grateful for friends and family, even if some of them still don't know whether I'm smart and understand what's going on. They don't really try to communicate with me, but I love it when my niece and nephews show real interest and talk to me. I have some great relationships with support workers who I know really care about me. They help me to know that I am sane and they help me be happy.*
>
> *Scott Clough*

One of the most critical deficiencies for people with disability – especially those living in group homes and institutions – is the lack of personal and meaningful relationships with others. If I can talk to support workers for a moment: you are often a significant person of influence in their life, much more so than they might be to you. It's important for parents to note that regular support workers are often your child's only peers, your person with disability's only 'friends' outside of family. This theme, therefore, is: 'Avoid isolation and encourage meaningful relationships. (Friends and family matter)'

Friends and family give life meaning. Interactive Carers in institutions, group homes, activity centres, sheltered workshops and any place that works with the disabled encourage family and friends to be involved with a client's life. They create opportunities for involvement and invite clients to special outings, creating opportunities to hang out with them – both at their house and out in the community. They're invited to events, meetings, goal-setting meetings and 'just because'. This, of course, is the ideal.

While I know of several group homes where the parents run the committee and organise special family days, making a huge effort to provide opportunities for family involvement, the day-to-day reality in many places is that visitors are not encouraged, particularly if you start asking questions or making waves.

Some families are not involved much or at all in their person with disability's life. This can be due to distance, age, the guilt of putting their loved ones into care, family dynamics, or a lack of understanding of their people with disability's ability to think, feel, love or communicate. The number of institutional residents in the special school I worked in who were 'wards of the state' – a term we no longer use but people still understand – was about two in five. It meant that their family members were either dead or had abandoned them.

It's problematic to discuss it, as I would not want to diminish the very real anguish that these family members may have gone through. I feel terrible that for nearly 10 years I only visited Scott once every 3–6 weeks – and even then it was usually just a brief visit. I was busy with my own life and I didn't feel very comfortable visiting his group home. I now find myself feeling terrible if I don't get to see him more than once or twice a week.

Involved family members know our people better than anyone. We usually care more than anyone – and, while every situation is different, families need to be given the due respect they deserve by providers. For people with disability who don't have an involved family, your relationship with them as a support worker is potentially a very meaningful one – if you foster it. You are sometimes their main source of connection to another person. Many support workers recognise this and cherish the relationships they create with their clients. After all, sometimes you are their only form of family.

Friends are a bit different, but equally important. Friends don't tend to share the history of trauma, guilt, righteousness, defensiveness and limiting beliefs that family can often be traumatised by. Friends, even extended family friends, can often see glimpses of possibility where family members and day-to-day carers don't.

Friends (and genuinely caring practitioners) can make a huge difference in anyone's life. Scott is so lucky to have practitioners like: Lyndon, whose friendship, intuition and immediately helpful therapy has been a huge help to Scott; Dagma, whose gentle counselling has been of enormous assistance; and the few medical professionals who actually do listen and are proactive with his medical needs. To you all: thank you.

For those with their people with disability living at home – those parents, children, siblings and grandparents caring for a family member who needs extra help – I salute you.

The chores of supporting them with substandard insufficient care can become exhausting, and the first thing that tends to wane is the fun stuff, the relaxed social times, and meaningful conversations. It can so easily become all about the practical day-to-day. Get support, ask for assistance.

If you've ever been on a commercial plane, you'll have seen the flight attendants give their safety speech. When they describe that oxygen masks fall from the ceiling in an emergency, they make a point of saying that you need to attach your mask first before helping others. Why? Because you are no help to others if you're incapacitated. You need oxygen (insert: sleep, nutrition, time off, financial advice, the occasional spa treatment and time with other family and friends) in order to do your job well.

The fundamental need to connect with others and not be isolated is the second part of this chapter about crucial, meaningful relationships. Even if the relationships are social ones rather than cherished ones, having connections with others who are friendly and encouraging ward against the perils of ostracism and isolation – a couple of the most insidious consequences of traditional disability care.

It has been documented in recent studies that being excluded and ostracised can threaten our psychological needs of belonging and having a meaningful existence. The impression of exclusion on our self-esteem is actually physically painful. Not only that, but it can have an effect on our rational thinking, physical function and our emotional behaviour.[28]

In the 1950s, university researcher Donald Hebb secured a $10,000 grant from the Canadian Defence Research Board to expand his research to human subjects on 'What Extreme Isolation Does to Your Mind'. The results were more dramatic than expected.

Depriving volunteer university graduate students of sensory input, he thought he would study the effects on their psychology for six weeks.

The majority of volunteers didn't last more than three days, and no one longer than a week. They were unable to think clearly about anything for any length of time. They were hallucinating and cognitive tests showed that their mental faculties had become impaired.[29]

So, while the experiment was extreme it was short lived. One can only imagine the effects of less extreme but long term (i.e. over years and decades) sensory deprivation, boredom and a lack of meaningful relationships on someone who already struggles with a physical or mental disability. It can be slow, well-meaning torture, and a self-fulfilling prophecy for those who propose that 'these people' will never cope in society.

In fact, being rejected by others can psychologically wound us more deeply than anything else. Several other studies confirm that loneliness isn't good for anyone's health. It increases stress hormone levels in the body and can lead to poor sleep, a compromised immune system and, in the elderly, cognitive decline. The pain of loneliness is a biological trigger, like physical pain or the ache of hunger and thirst.[30]

Anyone who's ever been bullied, had over-disciplinary parents or a vindictive teacher knows how negative words can affect us. Similarly, anyone who has spent a lot of time in their lives alone, or feeling invisible, knows what being ignored can do to the psyche. I know that many family members, support workers, practitioners and friends work very hard to instil in their person with disability that they are significant, unique and wonderful individuals. Even just my mum calling Scott her 'chosen child' means so much to him, I'm sure.

Interactive Carers see the potential in every client they work with.

Many people with disability form a strong bond with their favourite support worker because, apart from family, they are often the only other people that they spend real time with. This can be a privilege but it can also be a tricky relationship to navigate. I remember being quite young when I filled in for another support worker, working with a wonderful young man for a short time. Anthony used a wheelchair, was peg-fed (fed through a tube in his stomach) and communicated through a communication board, eye movements and cheeky smiles. I was instantly smitten with such a sweetheart, and we had a lot of fun together at his family home.

I only spent three days supporting him, over about a week, but he made it clear he had a crush on me. I carefully tried to step back, explaining that it wasn't appropriate for me to be anything but his 'carer'.

He took a while to feel his disheartenment and then started to cry – he spelled out on his board that he was lonely, asking, 'Who will love me?' Heartbreaking.

I wanted to tell him that everybody can find love, that he would find love and experience a relationship. Who am I to doubt that? But I had no words for him. I knew the odds of him finding someone were remote. It also made me think of Scott and all the other special friends I've made who happen to be disabled. To not ever experience true love or intimacy is a tough thing to live with. (I've since been challenged in recent years about this and now realise that, while it is still a rarity, it is possible for everyone to find someone special in their lives.)

I've seen Anthony a couple of times recently, as he moves in the same circles as my brother. I don't know if he's recognised me as that young lady who spent time with him all those years ago. He's probably had hundreds of support workers over the years, and while he made a real impression on me, perhaps he 'fell' for every female support worker! He still has that cheeky smile, and I wonder if he's found someone other than his family whom he can love.

Social inclusion can mean everything to those who don't otherwise have it. To feel like you belong in a community, and say hello to the people in shops and cafés, is very important.

People are usually willing to be friendly with someone with a disability, so getting to know the local shopkeepers, librarians, newsagent manager, postie, bus driver and neighbours is great to be part of your town.

Our friend Marlena Ketene doesn't speak and uses a wheelchair to get around. She wrote to me the other day that: 'The reality for me is I know EVERYONE in my neighbourhood and could walk down the road and get stuck on a gutter and still be okay.' She also added that, because everyone knows her, she feels that, 'If ever I was abused it would become clear to people.'

So a crucial component of the social model is for people with disability and their immediate carer/s to be social – not just with other carers, peers and family members, but inclusion with everyone in their community. So what does inclusion really mean? Haven't we stopped excluding people from schools and workplaces now? We have integration aids to help kids in schools. Isn't that inclusion? Well, yes, and no.

People tend to think there are two sides to the fence – either we are included or excluded – but it's more complex than this.

Several different support groups for people with autism have been strongly campaigning for a genuinely inclusive funding, education and living model. Before discussing that, let's talk about autism for a moment. Autism spectrum disorder (ASD) is a lifelong condition illustrated by difficulties in social interaction, using complex language and displaying repetitive interests and behaviours. ASD has a wide range of severity and varying characteristics, but all involve some form of neuro-developmental disability.

Two of the five different conditions along the spectrum are Asperger's syndrome (often having impaired social skills, few facial expressions, and limited interests) and autism (those with significant difficulty communicating and relating to other people, and repetition of certain behaviours). About 10% of people with autism are 'autistic savants', displaying extraordinary skills, often involving mathematical calculations, amazing feats of memory or artistic abilities.

Regardless of where on the spectrum they fall, people with ASD often have other symptoms as well, including learning disabilities, attention deficit hyperactivity disorder (ADHD), Tourette's syndrome, obsessive compulsive disorder (OCD) and depression.

Throughout history there has been a long list of significant people with autism spectrum disorder (ASD). While many are now deceased, the signs are clear and the people below are widely accepted as having been on the spectrum. They include Ludwig van Beethoven, Sir Richard Branson, John Denver, Albert Einstein, Henry Ford, Bill Gates, Vincent van Gogh, Abraham Lincoln, Michelangelo, Amadeus Mozart, Marilyn Munroe, Sir Isaac Newton, Steven Spielberg and Robin Williams.

Where on earth would we be without the impact of these extraordinary people in our world? They've changed history, invented the future, entertained us and helped us experience art and our humanity.

Finding ways to include any people with disability in society, particularly those with ASD, is not only possible – it makes social, community and economic sense.

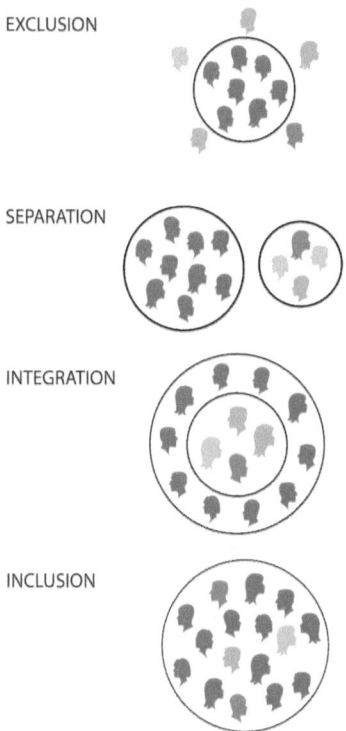

EXCLUSION

SEPARATION

INTEGRATION

INCLUSION

In general, institutional care is an example of complete exclusion. Special schools are an example of segregation. Having sporting teams for people with disability held during regular sporting meets is integration. And having people live, work, be educated and involved as individuals with regular people is inclusion.

In the pursuit of moving towards inclusion, transitions are often the most difficult time. Whenever your person with disability moves from one sphere to the next, there's likely to be an adjustment period. Anxiety can require support, but the pay-off is almost always worth it. Then we start the next transition. Depending on the condition, and the level of support, what can take hours or days for most of us dealing with change can take weeks, months or years for people with disability – but very real change does occur.

When we first began taking Scott out to theatre shows, movies and restaurants, he would get so excited that he'd squeal the place down. It sometimes became very embarrassing during a quiet moment in a play, or in a posh café – or he'd just fall asleep and we'd feel we had wasted our time and effort to take him somewhere. But we persevered and he matured, learning each time, and today we can take him to any show and any restaurant in the world with confidence.

In the Netherlands, the Coalition for Autism (Coalite Autisme) has demonstrated how inclusion not only is beneficial to the person with the disability, it makes social, community and economic sense too. It actually costs much more to society to segregate and exclude people with disability. Integration costs too, but you start to see a return on investment that is simply not there with the previous models. Inclusion costs the least to enact, and the benefit to society can be huge, as people with disability start to get jobs, earn their own money and contribute to society. Inclusion is not necessarily easy, but it makes economic, social, and moral sense for everyone in the community.[31]

Meaningful relationships – which we've established are crucial for all of us – happen more easily and frequently when the person is included in the community. The medical model's treatment of seclusion compounded the problems and ensured that the slow, meandering adjustment to social situations hardly ever took place. Now, with the social model moving to more inclusion in the community, people are being supported to reach their potential. It all depends on how you approach each individual case, and the continuous pursuit to inclusion, social interaction and meaningful relationships.

Imagine if your person with disability and their support worker both shared the same hobby, passion or skill. Wouldn't that symmetry add a whole new dimension to their relationship?

There's a website taking the disability world by storm, started by brother and sister team Jordan and Laura O'Reilly. They grew up with a brother with disability, and putting up with strangers in their house was part of their family life. Sometimes the support workers were a great fit for their brother and the family, but more often than not, they weren't. It got them thinking about how mutual interests can create a quick and genuine bond, and has more of a chance to develop into meaningful relationships.

So they created HireUp.com: 'Support workers who love what you love'. People with disability and their families can directly hire support workers based on their interests.[32] This online platform works well for anyone able to manage their own support workers, allowing them to find ones who share their interests. With the introduction of the NDIS across Australia, more people with disability have their own funding package so they can control who they hire.

It's like a springboard towards Interactive Care – having shared hobbies, skills or interests to accelerate interaction and meaningful relationships. As long as there are checks and balances to ensure the skills of the worker are there, and that the 'interest' list is verified, then it can be a fantastic way to set up a relationship for success.

For many people, the big challenge is that being able to live together as a family is what's essential – regardless of having a person who is aging or has a disability, injury or any other condition. Christos Iliopoulos is a philosopher from Melbourne who cared for his late wife Pamela for over 30 years as she battled with multiple sclerosis. He was so frustrated that the only options available for them seemed to be either to stay at home and receive inadequate care, or be relinquished to a nursing facility, or an institution away from loved ones.

Christos and his daughter Katherine have since invented Freedom Housing. The basic principle of this model is that four homes – in whatever individually unique configuration, size and style desired – are inter-connected at the rear through a 'key' building. The key may include a hydrotherapy pool, physiotherapy room, BBQ area, etc., and it provides an entryway for support workers to access each property, thus keeping the costs – shared between four households – down.

Elderly parents may live with their children, and children with disabilities may live with their parents. Individuals may live with friends their own age, or on their own if they prefer: whilst accessing the support they need, with as much (or as little) interaction with the other three households as desired. This is support with independence; it is inclusion in the community without the institutionalisation that comes with most supported accommodation options. Freedom Housing was the recipient of the 2013 Australian Human Rights Commission Business Award, and the first connected homes have now been constructed in rural Victoria.[33]

So, there are definitely new options emerging into the market. The problem is they are all private options, as the government struggles just to honour its commitment to the new NDIS, and is not even considering adding resources to the housing crisis for people requiring accessible, independent accommodation.

Christos is helping to address just one of the barriers to people with disability having lives that include family, friendships, love, fun, variety and genuine closeness. There are several barriers – but none that can't be overcome with thought, creativity, intention, care and a little bit of action!

Strategy Solutions

A. What can you as a family member or support worker do?

— There are many simple things that you can do to help facilitate or just allow for the possibility for those crucial, meaningful relationships to form, that make life worth living for all of us. Let's highlight perhaps the easiest, quickest and most significant one.

— In the movie *Avatar* the large blue people from Pandora have a special greeting: 'I see you.' It's meant to have been inspired by the Hindu greeting 'namaste'. To really see someone, to acknowledge the spark of humanity and uniqueness in them, is the ultimate way to honour and connect with them. That is our job when caring for anyone who can find themselves marginalised: the disabled, aged, infirm, injured, sick or homeless. The mentally ill, the new refugee and the dying. They all have a shining little light inside of them – and it's our job to find it, and then help them feel it and let them know that 'I see you'. That's how those crucial, meaningful relationships begin.

— Then there's the simple common sense strategies – like just getting out of the house! When you go up the street to a café, make a point of introducing your family member to the staff, so they can say hello and remember them the next time they visit.

— Go to pubs, festivals, outdoor community days, fun run walks and carols by candlelight events – and help strike up conversations with others there. Neighbourhood houses do cheap courses in a huge variety of activities. Going along to one of them with your person with disability helps to encourage meeting people, having conversations and building friendships.

— Play dates (or call them whatever you like for whatever age your person is) can be organised – people then have a quiet opportunity to slowly learn to communicate with each other. You can facilitate that as much as required, and feel safe to know they can just be alone with each other to find their own way and see if they want to spend more time together. The more people they meet, in a variety of settings – and variety of gender, age, able-bodied and disabled people – they more likelihood that some friendships will form and develop. It's all about practising the art of socialising, and becoming known in the community.

Additional Resources

— Link to two videos exploring Dr Emoto's work studying the effects of projected emotions onto water and rice:

1. ThinCube, 'Dr Masaru Emoto's Water Experiment - Words are Alive!', YouTube, <https://www.youtube.com/watch?v=au4qx_l8KEU>.

2. See Around Corners, 'Dr Masaru Emoto water experiment... scientific proof that the mind can effect the physical' [sic], YouTube, <https://www.youtube.com/watch?v=S7R-m5KJnYo>.

— Berson, S 2017, 'How often you hold your baby actually affects their DNA, Study Finds', Miami Herald, <http://www.miamiherald.com/news/nation-world/national/article186889938.html#storylink=cpy>.

Chapter 11

Support the Supporters!

> *We do need to make sure that the people who look after us are also being looked after. I've been there when a disability support worker who did a great job got into trouble, and I didn't like it. Especially when I know support workers who don't do a good job, and no one fixes the problem. They need better pay, permanent placements, (without all the odd shifts), and bigger thank yous.*
>
> Scott Clough

Throughout this book I've discussed the good and bad of support work. I've talked about the horrors of abuse and neglect, apathy, rorts, laziness, incorrect priorities, lack of knowledge and poor skills. But I've also discussed the heroes – the wonderful workers who give so much of themselves for their clients. The innovators, the intuitives, the guys who rock and the girls who roll!

This chapter is written firstly for support workers and service provider managers, to try to give some clarity and direction – from both a high-level and front-line level of any organisational workplace. Secondly, it's for family members, friends and advocates whose frustration with the system often gets directed at hapless support workers who are doing what they've been told to do – and truly don't often understand our explosions of irritation at every little thing we see wrong.

Our family flare-ups are usually a combination of seeing things that you (the worker) don't realise, combined with a sense of responsibility and self-reproach for not being diligent enough to prevent mishaps, and genuine concern from a historical context. You see, we've known them their whole lives. We've known them long before you – their support worker – came along. We've loved them and cried for them and had sleepless nights over them. Now we want to take them out for a meal and her shoes are on the wrong feet, his jumper is dirty and you haven't combed my mother's hair! Can't you see how upsetting this all is?

I don't mean to belittle families getting annoyed by the little things – because, as mentioned in touchpoints of care, these things are important. But perhaps the intensity with which we react at times can be felt by those at the brunt of our attacks as over-reactive and perhaps that nothing that you do as a support worker feels like enough. It can be a tough position to be in.

But the fact is that you're paid to look after the big thing and all the little things. If we don't tell you, we don't get to fix them, and you don't know our expectations. From our person with disability's perspective: we want everything we can get for them. We may have accepted their disability, but we don't have to accept less than exceptional levels of care for them.

> *'Your words, attitudes, and actions impact my life more than my disability.'*
>
> Kathie Snow, Author of Disability is Natural books and media, USA

I've been one of you. I know what it's like to be tired, stressed and overworked, with little to inspire you and far too few resources. I've seen hopelessly poor management, and know what it's like to work with difficult families, apathetic colleagues, draining clients and terrible work environments.

This last section – rather than being a theme of Interactive Care (as it's truly too important for that) – is essentially part two of this book. And while it may not require as many words as the themes, it's a crucial element in achieving any of this. If you're a disability support worker, I want you to know that everyone who is disabled – every family member of someone who is disabled, every practitioner, every friend and every other person – appreciates you!

I believe that one of the most important perspectives that will improve the lives of people with disability is how well providers look after the staff that do the lion's share of the work. Disability support workers deal with multiple clients and work casual shifts of all hours – for low pay, no job security, and with little reward or recognition. And the vast majority of them do it with huge smile on their faces, because they genuinely want to help people and overall do a great job. If we want them to do better, we need to treat them better.

The following five challenges highlight the need for both action and understanding to support the supporters:

1. Poor management destroys morale

We need higher quality management of disability support workers. That includes the entire gamut of providers: councils, charities, the big private providers, the small volunteer agencies, the religious groups, the one-to-one recruiters, and the online platforms. Whether you manage activity/work centres, supported accommodation or works in private homes, you have a huge responsibility on your hands, and I know it's not easy!

For more information on good management and leadership, go to 'What Managers Can Do To Create A Great Team' using the following link:

— 'Interactive Care – Resources', Mzuri Training, <http://www.mzuritraining.com.au/resources.html>

2. A lack of training belies the importance of the work involved

The standard Certificate IV in Disability is a foundation in practical and common techniques, OHS considerations, person-centric care, and good basic training for anyone entering this field. But there is no legal requirement for a disability support worker to have completed this training, and most providers either consider this qualification as 'desirable' or it's compulsory to have a certificate – but not necessarily in disability.

Most providers keep up with the legislative requirements of manual handling, first aid and other compulsory training, but with regards to leadership training, specific disability knowledge and keeping up-to-date with best practice in the field, most providers – and therefore support workers – can sometimes be sadly lacking.

We all know that we really learn our roles on the job, from those already in the job. The minimum standard of care is different for every provider, every manager – and, I submit, on every shift, depending on 'who's on'. This has got to change. Minimum standards of care must become the publically demanded norm across the board. Excellence has to become the minimum, giving people with disability a positive, stimulating environment, with choice, lifelong learning and connection to others.

3. Working conditions and career progression is important

An important element missing for those who want to make disability support their career is any form of career progression while still directly supporting people with disability. I've met several disability support workers who are studying in related fields, but there are so few courses specifically in direct care that if they want to study and progress in their career, they're virtually forced to move into aged care, social welfare or community services. This means that we lose the best, and are left with the rest. Again, support workers must have some sort of career progression if we want to attract and retain quality employees in this field.

And where is the built-in career progression for all the wonderful support workers out there? They deserve opportunities to learn, and – like in any other business – to get regular professional development. This means leadership, management and soft skill training, not just manual handling and other compliance training!

Support workers – like all of us – need reminding, and new practical ideas, of how to maintain a positive culture, what new resources are out there for themselves and their clients, and what's happening in their field in general.

Working conditions also leave a lot to be desired for many disability support workers. Lack of paid hours, decent pay, or workable routines destroys disability support workers' (and their family's) lives. Because the majority of support workers work casual hours, their income can be erratic and money is often tight. If we want support workers to do better – like teachers, nurses, and aged care workers – we need to pay them more.

I don't intend for this to be some aimless shout for something that will never come to pass. With fee-for-service, the NDIS, enterprise bargaining agreements and private contracting all occurring in this field, why can't we pay more qualified or experienced support workers more than the minimal wage? HireUp takes less commission than other agencies, so if you hire staff through them you'll pay less as a consumer – and if you're a disability support worker, you'll earn more.

One of the conditions of working in Christos's Freedom homes is that staff will have full-time permanent shifts and that there will be no uniforms for the staff. They need to be like a guest in the home – not in uniform like a nurse looking after a patient – and they'll have pre-arranged regular full-time shifts. This way, they have job security and regularity – and even more importantly, the clients will have consistency. They can plan activities ahead of time and it reduces not only their anxiety, but also enables everyone to manage risk more effectively.

The reality of the industry, however, is that conditions for support workers are moving in the opposite direction. Providers in Victoria have banded together and are currently trying to enforce a disability support worker collective agreement. This multi-employer Enterprise Bargaining Agreement would unite all the providers concerned and support workers could then easily work for any and all of the providers, accessing more work without requiring different contracts.

The proposed changes, however, seem to include lower hourly rates of pay, more travel (to different workplaces with different clients for the different providers), one week less of annual leave and an extension of eligibility for long service leave by 50%. If this comes to pass, then support workers will be even more disadvantaged than they are now, and none of this does anything to support, encourage or empower the very people we need to ably support our clients well. I hope the Health and Community Services Union (HACSU) and the Australian Services Union (ASU) can step up on this one!

4. Lack of recognition destroys morale

This fourth aspect of supporting the supporter is desperately in need of attention. People working in this field don't really have KPIs or sales targets, or really give a return on investment. They go full steam into challenging environments with average pay, little or no security and heavy-handed providers with untrained managers, looking after some of the most vulnerable people on the planet.

We know from recent research in business that what staff want in their work is to know that they're making an impact – that they receive some acknowledgement for the work that they do, in addition to deserved praise and recognition. They want flexibility and security – and the current system of rostered shifts, as with the retail industry, is rife with favouritism, nepotism and informal discrimination against people with diverse backgrounds or anyone who rocks the boat. (This last point was evidenced by all support workers who reported possible abuse occurring in their workplace refusing to give their names, out of fear of recrimination by their employer.)

There's little career advancement offered to most workers, and yet the strongest motivator for staff is a sense of progress. This could be interpreted as their own career progression, as well as what they sense they are achieving with their clients.

Each and every one of these aspects of workplace motivation are markers of 'touchpoints of care'. If we are demanding this standard of care from our workers, we must be modelling and providing the same care to them.

Dr Steven Covey, the old-school business guru who wrote the best-selling book *The Seven Habits of Highly Effective People*, said: 'Always treat your staff like you would have them treat your finest customers.' If you do, then you are setting up a culture of excellence, generosity, action and optimism. If you do not, then any positivity is purely opportunistic rather than genuine; there will be little loyalty or going above and beyond for clients, little sense of job fulfilment and a poor quality of life for the clients.

I have met support workers – with all different titles – who feel 100% supported by their provider organisation. I've heard them praise the directors and say how passionate they are, how loyalty is a two-way street in their company. I've heard it on the Mornington Peninsula with in-home disability support workers. I've heard it in Geelong where there are several in-home provider organisations with excellent workers whom I couldn't fault in any way. They insisted that they not only love their job, but wouldn't work anywhere else, as they trusted that their manager had their back.

This is so great, and I wish I heard it more often, but I don't. Until praise, recognition, support from managers and true leadership start becoming regular occurrences across the industry, we will always struggle to provide excellent care for people with disability, and abuse and neglect will continue to permeate in the darkness of burnt-out, resentful, untrained and apathetic workers.

5. Huge change creates huge stress

The work that the Department of Health and Human Services does in Australia is massive, and now with the NDIS, the changes have the potential to give people with disability more control over their lives than they've ever had before.

These changes, however, are shaking up the entire disability care system. Huge changes like this, even when for the greater good, can create havoc on disability support worker livelihoods – and, of course, lots of unwelcome change for their clients.

The massive upheaval in the council system alone is extremely concerning. Because I'm a leadership trainer specialising in government and health, I know that while 75 out of the 79 local councils in Victoria used to provide in-home, accommodation and day support for people within their constituencies, currently only a fraction of those 79 councils have made the commitment to becoming a preferred provider with the NDIS. Approximately 80% of the state that used to provide services soon will not.

Every one of the support workers who used to earn a living working with those councils will now have to change to other providers. While there should be plenty of work, there's no guarantee that they'll be working with the same clients, or doing similar duties or hours. That's very stressful and a huge upheaval for an entire sector.

Finally, there is that huge population of primary carers who look after their children or family members at home. It's these carers who survive with little government support and irregular respite care. They wouldn't change looking after their family member for anything, but they'd sure love some support. They get run-down, exhausted and deprived of the finer things in life – like having some time to themselves, paying the electricity bill, trying to organise a holiday for the family, or just affording decent food for the week.

Primary carers: you are the heroes of this nation. You have stepped up; you give love and guidance and support every day. You manage your household and supervise external support workers; you are disability workers yourselves as well as parents, cleaners, taxi drivers, employers, partners, researchers and innovative thinkers. Your need for praise, recognition, annual leave, a sense of progress, and professional development training are no less than a professional support worker. You need books like this, and live training, to re-invigorate, stay up-to-date, get ideas and model lifelong learning to your family. Seek it all out – you deserve nothing less.

The statistics are clear that primary carers survive with much less annual income than the average worker – and would cost the state billions of dollars each year if carers couldn't go on and had to ask the state to support their people with disability. With our aging population, this is a very real concern. We need to be making it not only liveable, but attractive to other family members to consider taking on this role. Government officials – state and federal – need to show some leadership on this issue and increase the carer's pension, providing funding for quality training and resources.

Parents of children with a disability, and family members caring for a person with disability: you need to put yourself first, on a regular basis, if you want to do a good job supporting your person with disability to be the best they can be. And remember the flight attendants giving their pre-flight safety speech: help yourself before helping others. You are no good to anyone else – and least of all the person with disability you're trying to support – if you are worn out, stressed out and burnt out.

Remember the process I gave the parents earlier in the book about dealing with frustrations? It goes for you too. Some families are difficult, some managers have been promoted to their level of (in)competence, and some colleagues need to find work better suited to their values! Sometimes they seem like the enemy!

The change that's required here is simple – but not necessarily easy. The crucial thing that will improve the lives of the people you support is to change your own mindset around the way you support them. By putting their needs first, and by thinking about things from their perspective – not just when it's convenient, but when it's inconvenient – can change everything.

Do you realise that, apart from family, you are often their biggest person of influence? What perspective are you coming from?

Little things that can make a real difference include:

— Don't be the centre of attention in the house! The residents are the focus. Yes, they want to hear about your day – and your new puppy or the movie you saw last night – but you're telling *them* about it, not the other carers, or going off on your own conversation with the client listening on without being included. They are the focus.

— Observe your client's privacy. If they get a phone call, and they don't require your assistance to communicate, leave the room to give them privacy. (Don't wait to be asked!) Give that respect to people in their own home. If they do require your help, then stay to assist, but everyone else can leave.

— Please support your clients to answer their front door. It's their house – not yours. Unless they specifically ask you to do so, or are physically incapable being moved, it's their role to welcome people into their home. Every time you answer the door, a tiny piece of ownership of their space and their independence is taken away.

— Please don't wear uniforms if you're working in someone's home. It's their home. You are not an official or a nurse running things. You are a guest in their home. Wear the same sort of clothing that they wear. As long as it's clean and respectful of their home-based culture, you will be appropriate.

— Have fun with your clients! I know you show affection and have a laugh when you can. I'm talking about showing initiative with fun, memorable activities – an impromptu indoor beach party in winter, a home-made pizza party on a Sunday afternoon, a maths competition, karaoke night, a paper plane making afternoon, a disco dance, or a board game challenge day!

As a final point on this chapter, on supporting the supporters, I just want to acknowledge the truly special support workers in Scott's – and therefore our family's – lives. People like Pauline, who was a member of our household for many years, Lyndon, a practitioner whose skill, gentleness and friendship have been very much appreciated. We've been blessed to have some wonderful people over the years – including our two currently most cherished disability support workers.

Olivia is a beacon of positive interactive energy, intuitive caring and lots of fun. She's the one who created the welcome home sign for Scott after his second trip to the USA. We all love you and thank you for your exceptional level of care.

And then there's Robert, who travelled with us to the USA, working crazy hours, when we were all dog-tired – especially during the 14-hour plane trips with no disabled bathroom! He coped with the dynamic between us family members, and did it all with grace, humour, professionalism and genuine friendship. His calm demeanour, knowledge and skill were also able to help Scott when he was in great distress and really needed it.

Your work is inspirational, and Scott, Mum, our whole family and I will be forever grateful.

Strategy Solutions

A. What can you as a family member do?

— I want to be absolutely clear to every reader that one of the most important steps to increasing the standard of care conducted by support workers is to **treat them better**.

B. What can support workers and their providers do?

— Managers: the most important step to increasing the standard of care conducted by support workers is to treat them better. Create a positive workplace culture, give the best ones job security, and stop employing the ones you know are not suited to the job. Increase the reward and recognition within your team.

— For a list of specific tasks an Interactive Care Manager does to lead a truly 'liveable workplace' with a positive culture that lasts, and get the best from their support workers, follow the link for a free PDF, 'This is good management and leadership': <http://www.mzuritraining.com.au/resources.html>.

C. What can we do as a movement, with and for people with disability?

— If you are a politician policy-maker, CEO of a service provider or anyone with any clout: please start making high-level changes to pay disability support workers what they're worth. We only get what we pay for – and these people are vital to the quality of life for some of the most vulnerable people on the planet – who are capable of contributing to our society in a very real way. Please support the supporters!

Additional Resources

— Disability is Natural, <https://www.disabilityisnatural.com/home.html>.

— 'Interactive Care – Resources', Mzuri Training, <http://www.mzuritraining.com.au/resources.html> to read the following linked article:

    1. Values in Action (PDF).

Chapter 12

Interactive Care Action

If you want to know how to make a real difference, check out the trainings.

Come and do the Interactive Care Course. I'll see you there!

Scott Clough

This book's main function was to outline the eight themes of Interactive Care – and to inspire everyone in this field to start to embody these themes in their everyday work, to effect attitudinal change.

'People may doubt what you say, but they will believe what you do.'

Lewis Cass

If you are a person with disability, or a family member, this book can guide you in what you can ask for from your support workers. For all managers of disability workers, this is your wake-up call to make life great for everyone by implementing Interactive Care improvements where they are appropriate. Everyone just needs to start thinking about what you could be doing differently, more consistently or more creatively.

And this is just the beginning. Where can you go to truly learn the answers, techniques and processes? How can you get practical experience working in an interactive way? Where can you learn with others in the field, practicing while you conduct research, have group discussions and question guest speakers?

As the director and lead facilitator of Mzuri Training, I have created a comprehensive, experiential, 12-day certificate course in Interactive Care. More about this later, but first – a question.

I am a trainer, a teacher and a coach. Yet I have heard many people with disability and family members state that the best support workers they've ever had didn't have any training at all! It's about the person and how intuitive and respectful they are, and whether they're a good fit for the client. So, why create a training course to help others become a high-quality disability support worker?

Because knowledge is necessary, training is relevant, and expertise is required when working with people with disability.

When finding new support workers for his wife, Pam, Christos from Freedom Housing would first give them the 'Pam Test'. This is when, instead of interviewing all of the applicants, he learnt to just let them spend 5–10 minutes with his wife first; she would give a secret thumbs up or down as to whether she would feel comfortable having them support her. This was the most important thing, then all other interviews and checks happened from there. He knew that they would then be best suited for the job – whether they had a certificate or not.

From that point on, this certificate course can take them to the next level and make this joint venture in support a long term prospect. To HR managers, directors and co-ordinators, it reminds me of the old business adage – better to train them and they leave, than we don't train them and they stay! Make training a priority, your reputation can depend on it!

To get academic for a moment – let's look at some studies done and their conclusions about the need for training. Bowman et al. (2010), Devries et al. (2014) and Sullivan et al. (2000) recommended the need for training staff in institutional settings to recognise signs of abuse, and also to respond to these signs – both by reporting appropriately and putting practices in place to safeguard the child.

Alriksson-Schmidt et al. (2010), Bowman et al. (2010) and Devries et al. (2014) focused attention on the need to increase staff knowledge and the capacity to respond appropriately. These authors specifically recommended training to be aware of factors that increase the risk of abuse, and protective factors and strategies to minimise occurrence.[34]

I believe that something significant has to happen if we're going to see any real change in the disability field. And I believe it starts with the people who provide daily care for the people concerned. We are still a far cry from the 21st century standard of support that we're capable of providing for people with disability. And we know it's possible because some are providing it.

It's time to support and train the managers, the parents and the workers. And not with online, bland or generalised theoretical workshops. For training about this topic to truly inspire people into action, it must be immersive, informative and experiential. Participants must develop skills (not just talk about them), conduct and present research, plan and conduct projects to enhance their client's skills, and develop their own personal mission statement.

The clarity and inspiration you can gain from the unique opportunities to discover true empathy, understanding and motivation – coupled with the practical skills, techniques and mindset to put new things into action – can make all the difference to your career, and their lives.

I'm reminded of the story told to so many by Loren Eiseley – a highly respected American anthropologist, scientist and poet – and used when starting a seemingly insurmountable task with little change of complete success. His version starts with an old man and a young boy. If I could be so bold, I'd like to tweak the characters for the purposes of this book.

> One day, a young girl was walking along the beach. It felt like her beach, as she lived nearby and liked to walk along it each morning for a few minutes before going to school. But this morning was a little different, as she saw a boy in a wheelchair enjoying rolling on the hard sand from the tide being out.
>
> As she walked closer, she could see him leaning down, almost falling out of his chair, and then getting up again and flinging his arms. He seemed to be doing it again and again. As she got closer, she noticed hundreds and hundreds of starfish that had washed onto the sand with the receding of the tide.
>
> 'What are you doing?' she asked him as he again flung his arms into the air.
>
> 'Hello. I'm throwing starfish into the ocean,' he matter-of-factly replied.

The little girl saw that the boy was indeed reaching down from his chair, carefully picking up any starfish he could reach, and throwing it back into the water with all his might. She had to ask: 'Why are you throwing starfish into the ocean?'

To this, the boy replied, 'The sun is up and the tide is going out. If I don't throw them in, they'll die.'

She looked around at all the starfish. He was right; they were all starting to dry out and change colour. They were all dying in the sun. 'But there's miles and miles of beach and there are starfish all along every mile. You can't possibly save them all. You're not going to make any difference.'

At this, the boy stopped for a moment, then bent down, picked up yet another starfish, and threw it with all the energy he could muster into the ocean. As it met the water, he turned to the girl, smiled and said, 'I made a difference for that one.'

Whether you end up doing things differently, more, or better as result of reading this book – I very much hope you do something. Go, make a difference.

Additional Resources

— Check out all of our free resources and links to further articles on the Mzuri Training website: 'Interactive Care – Resources', Mzuri Training, <http://www.mzuritraining.com.au/resources.html>

Afterword

You've made it through to the end of your first book on Interactive Care. Congratulations! I am truly humbled to have had you spend a few hours with me in revolutionising traditional disability care. I want you to know that these concepts and strategies really work, as long as you're putting in the actions and effort to really make it happen. Be kind to yourself, start small and build your success with your person with disability from there. Change can take time.

Now that you have collected this wealth of information and ideas, it's time to turn it into knowledge and experience. It's time to take action!

I encourage you to say 'yes' to every opportunity that comes your way to improve the lives of those in our care, and come from a space of service and gratitude every single day.

Best wishes,

Julienne

Next Steps

'Action is the foundational key to all success.'

Pablo Picasso

If you are a person with disability:

This book would be a great gift to give to all who support you! Know that you have the right to ask for the highest quality of support – and if they're not good enough, you can change them! Get in touch, as Scott wants to create fun meet-ups where we can tell our stories, listen to good music and have great food! Stay tuned for upcoming events.

If you are a family member/friend/advocate:

You can implement much of what's in this book. Remember, 'Action is the antidote to despair' (Joan Baez).

Scott would not have a method to communicate, high-quality medical care, weekly therapies, a wheelchair that suits his needs, international holidays, trendy clothes to wear or restaurant meals as regularly as he'd like – if it wasn't for his family taking the initiative to make these things happen. Providers usually do what they can, but are, by definition, limited in what they can provide.

Join our Facebook Group for all supporters in this field. (in Free Stuff)

Pass on this book to the managers at your provider organisations and let them know about what is possible.

If you are paid to support people with disability (disability support worker or any other relevant title):

After reading this book, pass it on to your manager!

Enjoy free access to all of the resources below.

Join our Super Support Workers Facebook group: <https://www.facebook.com/groups/429443650832414/>

Consider attending our workshops on Interactive Care, and becoming a certified Interactive Carer. (Any training you do can be claimed on tax if your provider doesn't fund it for you.)

<www.MzuriTraining.com.au/InteractiveCare>

If you are a manager in disabilities, aged care, nursing or education:

Pass this book on to your director!

Enjoy free access to the resources below for you and your staff. (All I ask is that you notify us about your use first, and acknowledge the source.)

Join our 'Magic Mzuri Managers' Facebook group: <https://www.facebook.com/groups/157734431606803/?ref=bookmarks>

Come to our workshops on Interactive Care, and consider becoming a certified Interactive Carer. Whole team workshops, special packages and deals are all available for Interactive Care training.

<www.MzuriTraining.com.au>

> *'You don't have to be great to start, but you have to start to be great.'*
>
> *Zig Ziglar*

About The Author

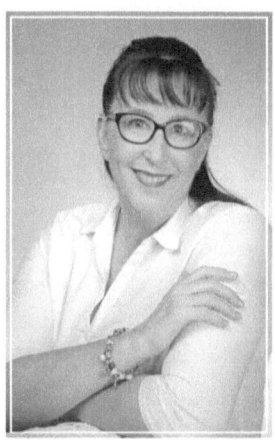

Director, author and lead facilitator, Julienne is the creative force behind (and face of) Mzuri Training. She is highly qualified (Advanced Diploma of Leadership and Management, Bachelor of Education, DISC Accredited, Cert IV Business Admin, Cert III Customer Contact) with nearly 30 years of experience creating and delivering exceptional teambuilding and leadership training throughout the Asia-Pacific region.

Julienne's dynamic, motivating and practical training builds on both her wealth of experience in the field and her expertise as an international speaker and trainer. She has trained many groups in the aged care, government, disability, health, education, hospitality and real estate fields in leadership, teambuilding, customer service, and presentation skills.

An 'Experiential Expert' in the field of disability, Julienne has worked in special developmental schools with severely to profoundly disabled adults, been a 'special home help' worker assisting children with disability in their homes, has been a companion to a people with cerebral palsy travelling throughout the world and educated staff on communication techniques for those without speech. She is also an advocate for her brother, Scott, who is a contributing author to this book.

Julienne is also an actress/singer – performing in the UK, Europe and Australia – a senior Drama/Theatre Studies teacher, playwright and director. She has lived in New York, London and Nairobi, and travelled throughout the USA, UK, Europe, Africa, Asia, India, Nepal, New Zealand and Australia. She currently lives by the bay in Melbourne and is a proud sister, daughter, aunty and friend.

Work With Julienne

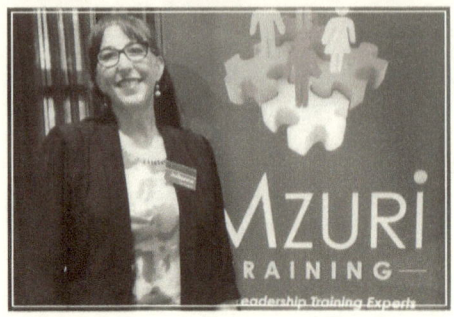

Julienne is a respected international speaker, trainer, coach, teacher and mentor. She lives in Melbourne, Australia but runs workshops interstate and internationally, and can coach clients anywhere in the world.

> 'Julienne is able to train from inexperienced managers to experienced managers in the same session using appropriate examples that connect with all participants. She has excellent technical knowledge, energy, heart and soul. When training, she demonstrates and role models exactly what she's training. She is real, confident, interesting and handles any difficult moments with grace and professionalism. She does not shy away from the "tough stuff".'
>
> Angela Anderson – Human resources manager (Brisbane, QLD, 2013)

Want a no-obligation 20 minute strategy session with Julienne, regarding training or coaching to make a transformation?

— As a disability support worker

— As a manager of staff in a group home or other facility that works with people with disability

Contact me now: <julienne@MzuriTraining.com.au>.

> 'The path to success is to take massive, determined actions.'
>
> Tony Robbins

Workshops

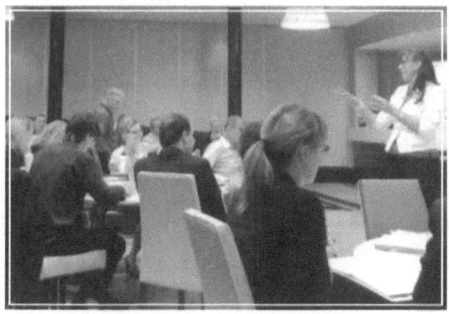

'Some great words of advice. We really need this form of training in this organisation as group cohesiveness is poor. Great, fun facilitation – well done on a lively presentation!'

Lisa Grassby – Disability support worker (Bairnsdale, VIC, 2017)

If you want something practical to start the Interactive Care conversation with your staff, download the Magic PDF – The 8 Themes of Interactive Care – for $5.95 from <http://www.mzuritraining.com.au/resources.html>.

Interactive Care: Breaking the mould of traditional disability care

½ day public workshops $97pp

Full day – onsite workshops $5,500 – for up to 30ptts

> 'Jules is an exceptional presenter. I would recommend everyone do these workshops it possible. They are extremely relevant.'
>
> Marge Amery – Office manager (Canberra, ACT, 2016)

See website for details: <http://www.mzuritraining.com.au/workshops.html>

Liveable Workplaces: Creating a positive culture that lasts

Full day onsite workshops – Australia/New Zealand-wide.

> 'Julienne, that was a great day, thank you so much. All of the staff enjoyed the presentation. A great day that was inspiring and energising for all staff.'
>
> Glenda McFee – Manager, disability care (East Gippsland, VIC, 2017)

<http://www.mzuritraining.com.au/creating-a-positive-culture.html>

Impressive Leadership Program

Mzuri Training's premier three-day leadership program, covering all main areas of leading others.

> 'Essential for every leader. A fun and energising way to learn. A great facilitator.'
>
> Sharon Perin – Manager (Adelaide, SA, 2016)

Download our detailed brochure: <http://www.mzuritraining.com.au/impressive-leadership-program.html>

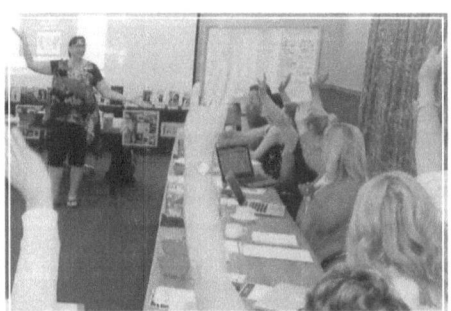

> 'An idea not coupled with action will never get any bigger than the brain cell it occupied.'
>
> Arnold Glasow

Interactive Care Certification

A premier certification for exceptionally trained, client-centred, highest quality personal support workers for people with a disability.

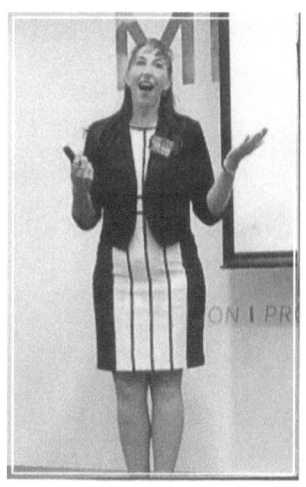

Interactive Care focuses on being a disability support worker, family carer or assistant for someone with a disability – particularly for those people with mobility issues and/or with little or no speech. It's a leadership, excellence, positive culture and customer service training program for workers in the disability field.

A 12-day program	run over 6 or 12 weeks (or retreat-style: 2 x 4-day live-in retreats)
6 theoretical days	workshop-style with activities, videos, and guest speakers.
6 experiential days	Interactive days in a facility. Skill practise with people with disability. Experience having a disability and be cared for – in a safe environment – with full debriefs afterwards. Set goals for yourself and your clients.
Assessments	Essential and optional reading, written assignments, practical assessments, research projects and presentations.

Why become a certified Interactive Care worker?

— To become a better disability support worker, and provide excellent service for your clients, organisations and families.
— To raise your professional profile, and the reputation of your organisation.
— To be able to educate your colleagues, family members and friends about what is possible.
— To become part of the movement to influence all the other support workers in the field, and be part of the Interactive Care revolution!

What's included in the course?

— 12 days of live, active training

— Guest speakers and multiple trainers

— Small group size for experiential days

— All essential resources provided

— Graduation dinner

— 12 months of group touch-base sessions.

Email <julienne@MzuriTraining.com.au> for a 20 Minute Strategy Session to find out if you qualify to attend the program.

Link to see detailed information: <http://www.mzuritraining.com.au/certification.html>

Packages Available

TEAM – one-day in-house workshop (three workshops for 25% off)

Three-Tier Interactive Care Package

Silver	Interactive Care Certification
	Twelve-day course
Gold	Silver, plus 6 x 1hr one-to-one
	Coaching and support sessions
Platinum	Both you and your team
	Gold x 1 + Silver x 2, with a team one-day in-house workshop
	Fully-refundable $500 deposit

I travel to speak and train this work all over Australia and internationally, so please get in touch with any questions or requests.

Julienne Verhagen – <julienne@MzuriTraining.com.au>.

Endnotes

1 Branley, A 2017, 'Group home 'hell': Open letter calls for royal commission into treatment of people with disabilities', Lateline, ABC News, <http://www.abc.net.au/news/2017-05-17/psychotropic-medications-in-group-homes-open-letter/8513664>.

2 Personal relationships, sexuality and sexual health policy and guidelines. Disability Services, Victoria, <https://providers.dhhs.vic.gov.au/sites/dhhsproviders/files/2017-11/personal-relationships-sexual-health-policy.pdf>.

3 'Final Report', Australian Government, <https://www.childabuseroyalcommission.gov.au/final-report>.

4 'Carers in Victoria – The Facts', Carers Australia – Victoria, <http://www.carersvictoria.org.au/Assets/Files/carers%20in%20victoria%20-%20the%20facts-2016-web.pdf>.

5 'Convention on the Rights of Persons with Disabilities', United Nations Human Rights, Office of the High Commissioner, <http://www.ohchr.org/EN/HRBodies/CRPD/Pages/ConventionRightsPersonsWithDisabilities.aspx>

6 'A Fairer Scotland for Disabled People' 2016, Scottish Government, <http://www.gov.scot/Resource/0051/00510948.pdf>.

7 Albrecht, G; Seelman, K & Bury, M (ed.), Handbook of Disability Studies, SAGE Publishing, <https://us.sagepub.com/sites/default/files/upm-binaries/26491_Chapter_1_Historical_Background_of_Disabilities.pdf>

8 'Adoption and Forgotten Australians', State Library Victoria, <https://guides.slv.vic.gov.au/adoption/forgottenAustralians>

9 Crossley, R 2010, 'Anne's Memorial Service', <http://www.annemcdonaldcentre.org.au/annes-memorial-service>.

10 'The social model disability', Centre for Independent Living, Northern Ireland (Head & Eastern Area Office), <https://www.cilbelfast.org/content/social-model-disability>.

11 '4430.0 - Disability, Ageing and Carers, Australia: Summary of Findings, 2012', Australian Bureau of Statistics, <http://www.abs.gov.au/AUSSTATS/abs@.nsf/allprimarymainfeatures/92730165AAFFD1FDCA25804F000F5F19?opendocument>

12 Wayland, S & Hindmarsh, G 2017, 'Understanding safeguarding practices for children with disability when engaging with organisations', Australian Institute of Family Studies, <https://aifs.gov.au/cfca/publications/understanding-safeguarding-practices-children-disability-when-engaging>.

13 'World Report On Disability' 2011, World Health Organization, <http://www.who.int/disabilities/world_report/2011/report.pdf>

14 Craven, Nick 2017, 'Genius inventor, 43, is helping scores of children by making state-of-the-art Spider-Man and Harry Potter-themed prosthetic arms in his garden shed', Daily Mail, <http://www.dailymail.co.uk/news/article-4525834/Inventor-Stephen-Davies-creates-prosthetic-limbs.html#ixzz5H0QxKqrD>.

15 Sarah Barton <http://www.disabilitybusters.com>.

16 Anne McDonald Centre, <http://annemcdonaldcentre.org.au>

17 Marlena Ketene, < http://www.marlena.com.au/interviews.html>.

18 John's Crazy Socks, <https://johnscrazysocks.com>.

19 'Our Year in Review 2016–17', Disability Services Commissioner, <http://www.odsc.vic.gov.au/wp-content/uploads/FINAL_DSC-2017-OYIR.pdf>.

20 2006, 'Protestors oppose sending Thai elephants to Australia', ABC, <http://www.abc.net.au/am/content/2006/s1656193.htm>.

21 Branley, A 2017, 'Group home 'hell': Open letter calls for royal commission into treatment of people with disabilities', ABC News, <http://www.abc.net.au/news/2017-05-17/psychotropic-medications-in-group-homes-open-letter/8513664>.

22 Disability Services Commissioner, 'Our Year in Review, 2016–2017', <http://www.oDisability Services Commissioner.vic.gov.au/wp-content/uploads/FINAL_DISABILITY SERVICES COMMISSIONER-2017-OYIR.pdf>.

23 ibid.

24 Branley, A 2017, 'People with intellectual disabilities locked away under cloak of suburbia', Four Corners, ABC, <http://www.abc.net.au/news/2017-03-28/people-with-intellectual-disabilities-locked-away-in-suburbia/8390350>.

25 STAR Institute for Sensory Processing Disorder, Non-verbal girl with Autism speaks through her computer 20/20 ABC News, YouTube, <https://www.youtube.com/watch?v=xMBzJleeOno>.

26 Khoo, I 2016, 'Carly Fleischmann Is All Grown Up With Her Own Talk Show', Huffpost, <https://www.huffingtonpost.ca/2016/05/03/carly-fleischmann-channing-tatum_n_9831922.html>

27 Carly Fleischmann, Carly's Café – Experience Autism Through Carly's Eyes', YouTube, <https://www.youtube.com/watch?v=KmDGvquzn2k>.

28 Williams, K D & Nida, S A 2011, 'Ostracism: Consequences and Coping', <http://journals.sagepub.com/doi/abs/10.1177/0963721411402480>

29 Mechanic, M 2012, 'What Extreme Isolation Does to Your Mind', Mother Jones, <https://www.motherjones.com/politics/2012/10/donald-o-hebb-effects-extreme-isolation/>

30 Burke, M 2009, 'Loneliness can kill you', Forbes, <https://www.forbes.com/forbes/2009/0824/opinions-neuroscience-loneliness-ideas-opinions.html#24ea12da7f85>.
31 Coalition for Autism in the Netherlands (Coalitie voor autism), <https://www.vanuitautismebekeken.nl>.
32 Hireup, <www.hireup.com.au>.
33 Freedom Housing, <http://freedomhousing.com.au/about_us.php>.
34 'Disability and child sexual abuse in institutional contexts' 2016, University of Sydney, p.46, <https://www.childabuseroyalcommission.gov.au/sites/default/files/file-list/Research%20Report%20-%20Disability%20and%20child%20sexual%20abuse%20in%20institutional%20contexts%20-%20Causes.pdf>.

www.ingramcontent.com/pod-product-compliance
Lightning Source LLC
Chambersburg PA
CBHW021112080526
44587CB00010B/488